Neuroplasticity

Your Brain and Its Strength, Capacity, and Intelligence

By Sally Stephens

Table of Contents

Chapter 1: The Hypothalamus *3*

Chapter 2: Tips for a Healthy Hypothalamus...*10*

Chapter 3: Is Your Brain Making You Fat? *17*

Chapter 4: Help Your Brain Get in Better Shape *25*

Chapter 5: About Neural Networks *31*

Chapter 6: The Creation of Databases...*37*

Chapter 7: Women's Brains *44*

Chapter 8: Social Cues *49*

Chapter 9: The Triggers of Libido: Men vs. Women *61*

Chapter 10: His and Her Brains at Work...*75*

Chapter 1: The Hypothalamus

A crucial to continual weight control is in knowing how to reset hypothalamus function preventing the body from trying to produce fat reserves. Our body has the lifesaving capability to save food energy as fat, in history when times were great and food was plentiful this functioned as a helpful purpose. Hunter-gathers often had times when there was little or maybe even no food at all, and these reserves of fat meant survival rather than hunger.

Now most people have lots of food available all of the time, so they no longer experience duration of feast or scarcity. For that reason, we really do not need large fat reserves any more. However, the hypothalamus has not progressed to recognize this situation. So, unless we can reset hypothalamus function with healthy eating that is thoroughly prepared, we will get fatter thanks to our body's old survival methods.

It is necessary to recognize that not only is the number of calories eaten essential, but so is the form of those calories. Fats, carbohydrates, and proteins are all used in different ways by our bodies, and there are distinctions in how the excess calories from those sources are stored by the body. By carefully picking the sources of our caloric consumption, we can reset hypothalamus responses to work in our favor rather than against us.

The hypothalamus gland lies within the brain. It carries out different functions, one of which is managing hunger. The hypothalamus develops signals that suggest when we are hungry and when we are satisfied. One problem that can happen is that the signal for being pleased has an integrated delay. So it can take up to 20 minutes right before the body recognizes that adequate food has been consumed. To try to compensate for this lag, you should focus on eating gradually so that you don't continue to eat after you are actually full.

Fat includes nine calories per gram, more than twice the 4 calories per gram found in proteins and carbs. Therefore, while any healthy diet plan requires some fat intake, you need to be extremely cautious to restrict the overall amount of fats you eat. What fats you do take in should be monounsaturated or polyunsaturated. Quality protein is always a really good choice, since it hinders hunger longer than carbs, is needed for healing and tissue structure, and is converted to fat extremely slowly.

Carefully picking carbs is the most crucial factor in re-training your hypothalamus from storing up fat. Simple carbohydrates, just like those found in syrup, honey, and sugar, take in into the body quickly. This results in a barrage of hormonal agents being released as a signal to the hypothalamus to begin hoarding fat. Complex carbohydrates, just like those found in fruit, veggies, and whole grain, take a lot longer to leak into the system. So they do not set off the fat-storing procedure. Putting less stress on your hypothalamus will keep you from saving up fat.

The way to evade the hypothalamus' impulse to store fat for lean times is to eat a healthy and balanced diet, tailored toward maintaining your existing weight. Such a diet consists of whole grains, intricate carbohydrates, healthy fats, and proteins but limits the consumption of easy sugars.

Hypothalamus - Role in Inspiration and Conduct

" Conduct is ultimately the item of the brain, the most mysterious organ of them all." Ian Tattersall (from Becoming Human.Evolution and Human Uniqueness, 1998).

The question of why we are encouraged to certain conduct's is maybe among the most essential in Psychology. Since Pavlov described conditioning in canines in his famous 1927 paper, scientists have pondered the origins of inspirations that drive us to action. For most of the early twentieth century, behaviorists like Watson & Skinner looked to explain behaviour in terms of external physical stimuli, recommending that learned reactions, hedonic benefit and support were intentions to generate a particular conduct. Nevertheless, this does not tell the entire story. In the last couple of decades, the school of cognitive psychology has concentrated on extra systems of inspiration: our desires according to social and cultural factors having an impact on behaviour. In addition, current advances in neuroimaging technology have allowed scientists an insight into the large complexities and modular nature of particular brain areas. This research has revealed that conduct's necessary for survival also have a fundamental natural basis.

The biological trigger for intrinsic behaviors like eating, drinking and temperature control can be traced to the hypothalamus, an area of the diencephalon. This book will check out the hypothalamic role in such determined behaviors. It is essential to note that a determined behaviour arising from internal hypothalamic stimuli is only one element of what is a complex and integrated reaction.

The hypothalamus links the autonomic nerve system to the endocrine system and serves many crucial functions. It is the homeostatic 'control center' of the body, keeping a well balanced inner environment by having specific regulative areas for body temperature, body weight, osmotic balance and high blood pressure. It can be classified as having three main outputs: the free nervous system, the endocrine system and motivated behavioral response. The main role of the hypothalamus in determined behavior was proposed as early as 1954 by Eliot Stellar who suggested that "the amount of inspired conduct is a direct function of the amount of activity in certain excitatory centres of the hypothalamus" (p6). This postulation has inspired a wealth of subsequent research.

Much of this research has been in the field of thermoregulation. The body's ability to maintain a stable inner environment is of vital significance for survivalas lots of crucialbiochemical reactions will only work within a narrow temperature level range. In 1961, Nakayama et al found thermosensitive neurons in the median preoptic location of the hypothalamus. Subsequent research revealed that stimulation of the hypothalamic area initiated humoral and visceromotor responses like panting, shivering, sweating, vasodilation and vasoconstriction. However, somatic motor reactions are also started by the lateral hypothalamus. It is far more efficient to move, rub your hands together or put on additional outfits if you are feeling cold. Likewise, if you are too warm you may get rid of some clothing or fan yourself to cool down. These inspired behaviours demonstrate that in contrast to a fixed stimulus response, motivated conduct promoted by the hypothalamus has a variable relationship between input and output. This interaction with our external environment might be a 'choice', however it is clear that the inspiration to make these choices has a natural basis.

The mechanics of thermoregulation can be clarified by what is sometimes referred to as 'drive states'. This is basically a feedback loop that is started by an inner stimulus which requires an external response. Kendal (2000) defines drive states as "characterised by stress and pain due to a physiological need followed by relief when the requirement is pleased". The process starts with the input. Temperature level changes are picked up from peripheral environments by thermoreceptive nerve cells throughout body which pick up both heat and cold separately. An electrical signal (the input) is then sent to the brain. Any divergence from what is referred to as the 'set point' - in this case a temperature of approx 37 ° - will then be recognized as an 'error signal' by interoceptive neurons in the periventricular area of the hypothalamus. Armed with these measurements and temperature signals being relayed from the blood, the hypothalamus then launches a proper mistake response. This includes motivating behavior to make a physical adjustment, e.g. to move around or eliminate surplus clothing in an effort to manage your temperature level.

This type of feedback system in the body prevails. Other systems needed for survival just like policy of blood salt and water levels are regulated in a comparable way. Nevertheless, the processes that encourage us to eat is far more complicated.

Humans have developed an intricate physiological system to control food consumption which encompasses a myriad of organs, hormonal agents and physical systems. Additionally, a wealth of speculative research supports the idea that the hypothalamus plays a crucial role in this energy homeostasis by activating feeding habits. Controlling energy balance is of vital significance and eating is primarily to preserve fat stores in case of food shortage. If fat cell reserves in the body are low, they release a hormonal agent called leptin which is found as a mistake signal by the periventricular region of the hypothalamus. This then promotes the lateral hypothalamus to start the mistake reaction. In this case, we begin to feel hungry which in turns mimics the somatic motor reaction by encouraging us to eat.

Since the hypothalamus also manages metabolic rate by keeping an eye on blood sugar levels, in theory we seem to have a comparable feedback loop to temperature control. However in practice this is not a reality. The main difficulty in keeping energy homeostasis is that inspiration doesn't rise up exclusively from inner natural impacts. Cultural and social aspects also play an important part in inspiration about when, what and how typically to eat. In western culture, public opinions to be thin can bypass the requirement to eat and in extreme cases like anorexia the drive state becomes reversed. The motivation is no longer to eat because they are hungry but is instead not to eat so they do feel hungry. This corruption of the benefit system is well recorded and is connected with deceptions of body image, an idea which is also linked to the hypothalamus and the parietal lobe. Issues can also take place if an individual receives over stimulation to eat. The occurrence of weight problems in today's society is testament to this fact.

Hypothalamus Summary

Anatomy and function
Hypothalamus diagram
Conditions
Symptoms
Heath tips

What is the hypothalamus?

The hypothalamus is a small region of the brain. It's located at the base of the brain, near the pituitary gland.

While it's very small, the hypothalamus plays an important role in tons of important functions, consisting of:

launching hormonal agents
regulating body temperature level
preserving everyday physiological cycles
controlling appetite
handling of sexual behavior
regulating psychological responses

Anatomy and function

The hypothalamus has 3 main areas. Each one includes different nuclei. These are clusters of neurons that perform essential functions, like releasing hormones.
Anterior area

This location is also called the supraoptic area. Its significant nuclei include the supraoptic and paraventricular nuclei. There are several other littler nuclei in the anterior area as well.

The nuclei in the anterior region are mostly involved in the secretion of different hormones. Many of these hormonal agents connect with the nearby pituitary gland to produce additional hormones.

Some of the most essential hormonal agents produced in the anterior area consist of:

Corticotrophin-releasing hormonal agent (CRH). CRH is involved in the body's response to both physical and psychological tension. It signifies the pituitary gland to produce a hormonal agent called adrenocorticotropic hormone (ACTH). ACTH sets off the production of cortisol, an vital tension hormone.

Thyrotropin-releasing hormone (TRH). TRH production stimulates the pituitary gland to produce thyroid-stimulating hormonal agent (TSH). TSH plays an important role in the function of tons of body parts, such as the heart, intestinal system, and muscles.

Gonadotropin-releasing hormonal agent (GnRH). GnRH production causes the pituitary gland to produce crucial procreative hormonal agents, like follicle-stimulating hormone (FSH) and luteinizing hormonal agent (LH).

Oxytocin. This hormone manages tons of crucial behaviors and feelings, like sexual arousal, trust, recognition, and maternal conduct. It's also involved in some functions of the reproductive system, such as childbirth and lactation.
Vasopressin. Also called antidiuretic hormonal agent (ADH), this hormone controls water levels in the body. When vasopressin is released, it signifies the kidneys to take in water.

Somatostatin. Somatostatin works to stop the pituitary gland from releasing certain hormonal agents, including growth hormonal agents and thyroid-stimulating hormones.

The anterior region of the hypothalamus also helps manage body temperature through sweat. It also keeps body clocks. These are physical and behavioral changes that occur on a daily cycle. For instance, being awake during the day and sleeping at nighttime is a circadian rhythm associated to the presence or lack of light.
Middle region

This area is also called the tuberal area Its significant nuclei are the ventromedial and arcuate nuclei.

The ventromedial nucleus helps manage appetite, while the arcuate nucleus is involved in launching growth hormone-releasing hormone (GHRH). GHRH stimulates the pituitary gland to produce development hormonal agent. This is responsible for the growth and development of the body.

Posterior area.

This location is also called the mammillary region. The posterior hypothalamic nucleus and mammillary nuclei are its main nuclei.

The posterior hypothalamic nucleus helps control body temperature level by triggering shivering and obstructing sweat production.

The role of the mammillary nuclei is less clear. Doctors actually believe it's associated with memory function.

Hypothalamus conditions

When the hypothalamus doesn't work correctly, it's called hypothalamic dysfunction.

Some things can cause hypothalamic dysfunction, including:

head injuries
certain genetic disorders, just like development hormone deficiency
abnormality involving the brain or hypothalamus
cancers in or around the hypothalamus
eating conditions, such as anorexia or bulimia
autoimmune conditions
surgery involving the brain

Hypothalamic dysfunction contributes in a lot of conditions, consisting of:

Diabetes insipidus. If the hypothalamus doesn't produce and launch enough vasopressin, the kidneys can remove way too much water. This triggers increased urination and thirst. Unlike people with diabetes mellitus, people with diabetes insipidus have stable blood glucose levels.

Prader-Willi syndrome. This is a rare, acquired condition. It triggers the hypothalamus to not sign up when someone is full after eating. People with Prader-Willi syndrome have a constant desire to eat, increasing their risk of weight problems. Additional symptoms consist of a slower metabolism and decreased muscle.

Hypopituitarism. This disorder happens when the pituitary gland doesn't produce adequate hormones. While it's generally caused by damage to the pituitary gland, hypothalamic dysfunction can also trigger it. Many hormones produced by the hypothalamus directly impact those produced by the pituitary gland.

Symptoms of hypothalamic conditions

Hypothalamic conditions can trigger a variety of signs. Which signs you might experience depend upon the part of the hypothalamus and types of hormonal agents included.

Some signs that could signal a hypothalamus problem consist of:

unusually high or low blood pressure

body temperature changes
unusual weight gains or loss
changes in hunger
sleeping disorders
infertility
short stature
postponed start of puberty
dehydration
regular urination

Chapter 2: Tips for a Healthy Hypothalamus

While some hypothalamus conditions are unavoidable, there are a few things you can do to keep your hypothalamus healthy.

Eat a balanced diet plan
While eating a balanced diet is important for each body part, it's particularly crucial when it concerns the hypothalamus. A recent study in mice found that eating a high-fat diet plan led to inflammation of the hypothalamus.

Another study in mice found that a high-sugar diet also triggered swelling of the hypothalamus. To decrease your danger, ensure you'reaware of how much sugar you take in daily.

Get enough sleep

A 2014 study found that sleep deprivation was connected with hypothalamic dysfunction in rats. Besides, scientists involved in the research study suggest that sleep deprivation may increase someone's risk of neurological diseases.

If you have a hard time sleeping, try these 10 natural solutions to help you sleep and keep your hypothalamus working effectively.

Does the Hypothalamus Regulate Weight Loss and Gain?

There are a lot of things that lead people to gain weight along with reduce weight. The primary cause of weight gain is unhealthy eating and lack of exercises. The body gains weight when the amount of calories introduced to the body is more than the amount of being used up by the body. Weight-loss is the precise opposite, when the amount of calories taken in is less than what is being consumed by the cells. This happens when the body under goes intense workout and taking in much healthier foods.

For all these changes to occur, a mix of several factors inside our bodies need to collaborate. When one is feeling starving, you will hear a grumble from the stomach. The hypothalamus is what triggers the roar. Hypothalamus is a small part of the rear of the brain that manages the majority of our emotions from thirst, hunger, taste and so on.

Hypothalamus can help you reduce weight in that any time you feel starving you eat the right kind of food. If you feel starving very quick you should ensure that you have within your reach food that contains a ton of fibers like oat meal and fruits. These foods with fibers are not easily absorbed for that reason stay longer in the digestive system giving you the impression you are full all the time.

The hypothalamus also helps you eat less in that whenever you eat slowly it takes time for that reason the hypothalamus informs you that you are full. Develop the practice of eating should also begin eating gradually if you want to slim down. This is because your body takes twenty minutes to notify you mind that you are full.

The hypothalamus spots any irregular changes in the body and is able to react accordingly to effect the essential changes that will return the body to its regular condition. It will keep in mind if you are eating healthily or unhealthy or introduce any foreign substance into your body like drugs. There are sensory organs all around the body that find changes in the glucose and water level in the body. Whether there is a rise or fall, and sends signals to the brain which triggers you to crave for water if the water levels in the body are low. The exact same occurs with glucose so that you want to eat something sweet, at this time instead of eating candy and other unhealthy sugary stuff; you can choose to eat a meal or a natural source of sugar.

Normally, the hypothalamus helps in managing weight, by the emotions that it impacts. When you get these emotions of cravings and thirst you know what is going on in your body and for that reason you can react by consuming healthy. However, when you feel hungry and you let your hunger lead you, your body will just follow what you do and you will gain weight. You should eat healthy, slowly and in moderation when you are hungry.

How to Recognize Pituitary Gland or Hypothalamus Damage After a Head Injury

Head Injury and Hormone Dysfunction

Terrible brain injury, also called TBI, can harm the hypothalamus and pituitary gland. Located at the base of the brain, they control our hormones and can release insufficient or increased hormonal agents when damaged, so interfering with the body's ability to keep a steady inner environment.

When pituitary gland damage causes decreased hormonal agent production, the condition is called hypopituitarism and was initially reported practically 100 years ago. Originally believed to be an unusual incident, current research on adult survivors of severe brain injury, now report the occurrence of pituitary hormone shortages to be between 23% and 69%.

Signs and assessment

The majority of people's hormonal agent levels are seriously affected in the early phases after distressing brain injury, even if the pituitary is undamaged. This makes pituitary damage tough to identify and whilst later in the healing process it may become clear that some signs are caused by hormone changes which can be tested, there are currently no clear guidelines for the evaluation and treatment of pituitary function after brain injury.

The effects of pituitary and hypothalamus injury differ just because of the different hormonal agents which can be impacted and some signs are also comparable to the more typical effects of brain injury, which is another reason why the issue is not easily diagnosed.

Overlapping symptoms are:
Anxiety
Impotence and altered sex drive
State of mind swings
Fatigue
Headaches
Visual disruption

Other signs include:
Muscle weakness
Decreased body hair
Irregular periods/loss of regular menstrual function
Reduced fertility
Weight gain
Increased cold level of sensitivity
Irregularity
Dry skin
Pale appearance
Low blood pressure/dizziness
Diabetes insipidus

Whilst each sign may be brought on by a modification in the level of a particular hormone produced in the pituitary gland, there are a lot of possible reasons for all of these symptoms, so a thorough assessment is needed right before a firm diagnosis can be made.

Treatment

Early on, hormonal problems can cause neurogenic diabetes insipidus, which is characterised by increased thirst and extreme production of dilute urine. This is because of a decrease in a hormonal agent called vasopressin (anti-diuretic hormonal agent) and is treated by administering desmopressin and changing lost fluids.

In the later phases, if hypopituitarism is validated, hormonal agent replacement treatment might be used to restore typical hormone levels, to help manage the symptoms. There are different treatments readily available, depending upon the particular hormonal agents involved and the nature and degree of the symptoms.

The assessment and treatment of hypopituitarism after brain injury is an intricate procedure and just like any treatment, you should talk about the advantages and disadvantages with your physician right before making any choices.

Further info

The full extent of hypopituitarism after brain injury is unknown, whilst it seems to occur primarily after serious brain injury some research studies have shown that pituitary gland damage might also occur after obviously small head injuries. However, lots of the symptoms can be caused by damage elsewhere in the brain, and if this is the case treatment for pituitary dysfunction will not work.

If you believe signs of hypopituitarism, or any other hormone condition, you should speak to your GP who, if they feel it appropriate, may refer you to an endocrinologist who can run a range of hormonal agent level tests and even a scan, to try to find damage to the hypothalamus or pituitary gland.

The Hypothalamus in BBT Limitations

The hypothalamus is a small gland found at the base of the brain, which basically operates as a thermostat for procreative hormonal agents. It controls the levels of some hormones produced by offering responses to and stimulation of the pituitary gland.

How does the hypothalamus work?

The hypothalamus produces gonadotropin-releasing hormonal agent (GnRH), which signifies to increase or reduce hormone production throughout the very first stage of a ladies's ovulatory cycle. In the feedback reaction, the pituitary boosts FSH production that then triggers hair follicle production in the ovaries. The production of estrogen is then accomplished as the roots enlarges. As estrogen levels increase, the FSH levels eventually reduce. Once the hair follicles are mature, the hypothalamus signals a spike in luteinizing hormone (LH), which causes ovulation 36 hours later. If something within this course is irregular or missing, and the procedure of ovulation doesn't take place, infertility will result.

Irregular ovulation can be due to many factors, but most regularly is secondary to the failure of the ovary to produce a roots that ovulates. Anovulation happens when the ovaries cannot launch eggs for fertilization. Although this is a natural consequence of aging associated with menopause, it might take place previously in some ladies.

Some factors in irregular ovulation are:
1. Hyperprolactinemia - abnormally raised prolactin levels. This might be because of a little tumor on the pituitary and might need medications and/or surgery.
2. Thyroid dysfunction - hyperthyroidism or hypothyroidism. Thyroid levels can trigger irregular ovulation. Medications can be used to deal with thyroid dysfunction.
3. Adrenal disorders. Androgens are male hormones, such as testosterone, produced by the ovaries and adrenal gland. High levels might result in oligo-ovulation.
4. Ecological factors like contamination, radiation, etc.
5. Extreme exercise, weight problems, and/or tension

Fertility treatments are available for such cases. In these circumstances, it is presumed that the fallopian tubes are still open, unless the client has had a tubal ligation surgical treatment. A unique test called a hysterosalpingogram can be done to make certain that the fallopian tubes are open. If the client has had a tubal ligation, she would need to have a tubal turnaround carried out to open the tubes again. Any patient who will be going through a tubal ligation turnaround would take advantage of a hormone examination right before the tubal turnaround surgical treatment to guarantee that once her tubes were reversed, she would not have infertility from a hormonal issue.

Sleep Hyperhidrosis and Fevers

While it may appear obvious, a typical reason for night sweats is a basic fever. However, even a basic fever can be alarming if left unattended.

But why does having a fever have to make us sweat? To comprehend this, we have to understand our inner thermostat. Our inner thermostat is a part of our brain called the hypothalamus.

The Hypothalamus: The Human Thermostat

Our hypothalamus might be reasonably small compared to the remainder of the brain, but this little area of cells is a key junction point between our nervous system and endocrine system. These two essential natural systems come together in the pituitary gland at the base of the hypothalamus.

Unfortunately, our hypothalamus can be susceptible to various impacts both inner and external. Anytime something causes a chemical imbalance or hormonal shift in our bodies, the hypothalamus can react in an unexpected way. Hence potent drugs and even foods may trigger it to respond erratically. It also helps us comprehend why the sharp hormone shifts that happen during menopause can cause hot flashes and night sweats.

Adjusting the Thermostat for An Infection

One of the core functions of the hypothalamus appears to be to manage our temperatures when an infection is present. When a foreign germs or infection is spotted in our bodies, our hypothalamus raises our core temperature level to help our bodies fight off that bacteria or infection. If you experience the chills or the shakes, this is often a side-effect of our hypothalamus attempting to regulate our nervous system and gland in an optimal style to combat off the infection.

Once the hypothalamus has identified that your immune system has won the fight with the bacteria, it begins to set your core temperature production back to its baseline temperature level. To release the excessive heat and bring your temperature down, it kicks in some natural functions. One our bodies best tools for dissipating heat is through sweating.

Confusing the Thermostat with Medications

Medicines that lower our body temperature levels-- typically referred to as antipyretics-- often interrupt appropriate signaling between our immune system and our hypothalamus. This leads to sudden shifts in our body temperature level. When such unexpected, external sources of influence impact the hypothalamus, our hypothalamus usually reacts by triggering heavy sweat much like it would if we were recuperating from a high fever.

As you can see, periodically our body naturally incurs night sweats while recovering from or adapting to a fever. And sometimes our body is reacting to the drugs we might have brought to deal with the source of that fever. But in both cases, the source of the night sweating is our hypothalamus doing its finest to regulate our endocrine and nerve systems to safeguard our present condition.

The Biology of Sweating While Sleeping

If you're concerned about sweating while sleeping, it will help you to understand why your body perspires when it does. Once you understand what's going on when you perspire in the evening, you will have a better idea what steps to take to stop the sweat.

Your Internal Thermostat

All of us have an inner thermostat. It is almond-sized and it sits at the top of your brain stem. It is called the hypothalamus.

The hypothalamus carries out crucial functions in the free nervous system. It controls your sense of cravings and thirst, your sleep cycle and most appropriate to this conversation, your body temperature level.

This internal thermostat carries out thermoregulation by receiving signals from thermosensitive neurons in your brain and temperature receptors in your skin.

Confusing Your Hypothalamus

Regrettably, the hypothalamus can be susceptible to a number of external impacts, most often uncommon hormone fluctuations and medications (both non-prescription and prescription). When your hypothalamus receives blended signals from these sources, it sends out blended signals to the rest of your nervous system.

This is why menopause triggers hot flashes and why so many medications have sweating while sleeping as a side-effect.

Common targets of these blended signals from your hypothalamus are your gland.

Gland

The body functions eccrine sweat glands all over the body in its skin. While these glands excrete water, electrolytes and toxins, their primary function is to perform thermoregulation-- to put it simply, to control your body temperature. So when you are perspiring, your hypothalamus is telling your sweat glands to produce an evaporative cooler on your skin.

Human gland are quite basic body parts. They only do as their told by your hypothalamus. So it is important to recognize that when you perspire, you are doing so as your brain has told your gland to activate.

Negotiating with Your Hypothalamus

So if you really want to stop sweating while sleeping, you need to determine why your brain is telling your gland to trigger at night while you are asleep.

If your hormones are to blame, research what foods and supplements may mediate your hormonal fluctuations. If you are taking a medication with night sweats as a side-effect, you may consult your medical professional about adjusting or changing your medications.

If it is just your skin sensing units telling your brain you're hot, then you really need to take steps to better control variables like your sleep environment and your diet to keep yourself cool during the night.

Chapter 3: Is Your Brain Making You Fat?

The words are most likely crossing your mind right now. "Sure genius, my brain lets me know I really need to eat, so that's what I do (and probably more regularly than I should). Then bingo. the love handles, thunder thighs, and the ever notorious muffin top we have all grown to really love, right. Very wrong. you would never actually know it, but there's a little area in your brain that is perhaps sending messages throughout your body to not just eat processed food, but eat tons of it.

What on the planet is this little piece in my brain and how do I get it eliminated you might be thinking? The location is known as the hypothalamus gland, unfortunately getting it got rid of is not the answer because doing that might lead to a lot more problems. For example, getting it eliminated could lead to death. It holds true, and though the size of a peanut, this gland is a really fundamental part of your brain that is crucial to the performance of your body. This gland when skewed (which is actually quite simple) can add to many issues, among which could be some not so ideal lumps in areas they should not be in.

Why you have the hypothalamus and its function is to connect the endocrine system up with the nerve system. The endocrine system which is a mix of some glands and organs, like the thyroid, adrenals, pancreas, pituitary, and some other ones is the system that controls most of your weight. Issues with the hypothalamus can wreak havoc on your entire system which can increase food yearnings, slow your metabolic process, and trigger your body to keep what are called "safe fat reserves".

The body stores these so called "protected fat reserves" in the most problematic areas and thinks about fat in those parts to be kinds of fat that is last in line to be burned up. This is the reason that regular diets that advise you to reduce calories or restrict certain foods don't work. Another intriguing point is that because the hypothalamus gland mainly manages the bodies weight set point, it clarifies why when such diets are completed many people gain back the weight that they had loss throughout the diet.

Why then does a normal appropriately functioning gland develop into something that becomes damaging to your health? There's many reason why this can happen, either straight of indirectly the gland can become overworked is a main reason. Too call several methods the gland can become overworked we can begin with the fact that the majority of us lack simple workout daily like walking, having a clogged up colon, not taking in the right types of nutrients, eating exceedingly improved foods that have all kinds of chemicals and growth hormonal agents in them. With time and especially the last few decades the problem has ended up being progressively and undoubtedly worse with the tons of changes to our food system being designed in a way to make severe profits, and not so much extremely healthy food.

With much thanks, like many other sicknesses you can get, the gland behind all of it can slowly be brought back to correct performance. Because the food we eat is a main reason regarding why the gland ends up being problematic, a basic change to organically grown foods and avoidance of the fine-tuned and overly processed foods can have a huge assisting effect. It might also be valuable to think about an easy cleanse of the liver, colon, and detoxing candida and parasites.

Simple exercise routines like walking or riding a bike each day will also help significantly. What you should aim to do is to reset your hypothalamus gland which is dealing with the cause not just a sign. This certainly will take a lot of work as tons of mental adjustments are necessary, yet it's possible. This one step in the right direction could lead you down a course of weight reduction and better life long health.

6 Natural Ways to Boost Hypothalamus Function

The hypothalamus is a vital part of the human brain and is usually considered the nerve center for the majority of hormonal agents. Its working relationship with the pituitary gland as well as the adrenal glands affects our nerve systems in addition to our endocrine systems. But what does the hypothalamus do exactly? For starters, it plays a part in our calorie intake, weight regulation and temperature. I m sure you'rebeginning to get the picture that, even if you weren't already familiar with hypothalamus function, it plainly is necessary to human existence.

The hypothalamus lies deep within the brain, just above the base of the skull. Its primary general function is to control homeostasis of our bodies. To put it simply, it helps keep the human body in a constant, consistent state. When the hypothalamus doesn't function properly, this shakes off the functioning of the pituitary gland. But it doesn't stop there since the pituitary gland manages the adrenal glands, ovaries, testes and thyroid gland. So when hypothalamus function isn't right, there are a ton of other things impacted that are all important to health.

Recent research even shows that many elements of aging are controlled by the hypothalamus. Studies give hope to the possibility that we might be able to change signaling within the hypothalamus to slow down the aging process and increase longevity. Let's have a look at precisely when and how the hypothalamus can impact our health and how we can naturally boost the function of this underrated gland.

These are the best ways:
1. Increase Chromium Consumption

Chromium is a trace mineral needed by the body in percentages for healthy functioning. The hypothalamus is incredibly important, a main part of the free nerve system that helps controls body temperature level, thirst, appetite, sleep and emotional activity. Research studies have linked chromium with much healthier hypothalamus function. Research suggests that it can help keep the hypothalamus in a more younger state, better regulate hunger in senior adults and stop negative effects on brain nerve cells triggered by aging.

Below are 10 of the best food sources for obtaining more chromium naturally through your diet:

Broccoli
Potatoes
Garlic
Basil
Grass-fed beef
Oranges
Turkey
Green beans
Apples
Bananas

You might want to consider supplementing with chromium, but the benefits of taking chromium supplements are still rather questionable and questioned by some medical specialists since studies to date program combined actual results. If you can, it's finest to get chromium from natural foods.

2. Usage Essential Oils

Vital oils of frankincense and myrrh do not just have extremely lengthy histories of usage going back to biblical times they've also been shown to enhance brain health. Two main active substances called terpenes and sesquiterpenes are found in both frankincense and myrrh oil. Both of these substances have anti-inflammatory and antioxidant effects on the body.

Sesquiterpenes have the ability to cross the blood-brain barrier and stimulate the limbic system of the brain and other glands promoting memory and launching feelings. Sesquiterpenes have been found to increase oxygen around receptor sites near the hypothalamus, pineal and pituitary glands. Sesquiterpenes also particularly have a result on our psychological center in the hypothalamus, helping us stay calm and well balanced.

There are tons of ways to incorporate frankincense and myrrh into your daily life. You can diffuse the important oils, inhale them straight from the bottle, or you can blend them with a carrier oil like jojoba and use the mixture directly to the skin.

You can try making Homemade Frankincense and Myrrh Cream, which is a remarkable way to quickly include both of these essential oils into your daily regimen.

3. Try Vitex (Especially If You'rea Female).

Vitex, also known as chaste tree berry, is an organic supplement highly well-known for its capability to help balance female hormonal agents. The medical ability of chaste berry to positively impact hormone health concerns seems derived from dopaminergic substances present in the herb. How exactly does vitex encourage hormone balance? While it doesn't supply hormones to the body, it does act directly on the hypothalamus and pituitary glands. For women, it increases luteinizing hormone, modulates prolactin and aids in the inhibition of the release of follicle-stimulating hormone, which all help cancel the ratio of progesterone to estrogen, somewhat raising the levels of progesterone.

If you experience infertility and/or PCOS, vitex can be especially practical. Vitex or chaste berry is readily available in various types in your regional health shop or online. The dried, ripe chaste berry is used to prepare liquid extracts or strong extracts that are put into capsules and tablets. If you'renot a fan of pills or tablets, then the liquid extract is a great choice. You can also easily find vitex in tea form on its own or integrated with other herbs that promote hormone balance. You can also order the dried berries and make your own cast in the house.

4. Eat Healthy Fats.

In addition to vitex, there are lots of other natural ways to balance your hormonal agents and accomplish better hypothalamus function. Developing hormonal balance in your body has a direct positive effect on the function of your hypothalamus along with your pituitary gland. Among the best methods to stabilize your hormones through your diet is to regularly consume healthy fats.

Cholesterol and other fats play a basic part in structure cellular membranes and hormones. Certain kinds of fats, consisting of cholesterol, also act a lot like anti-oxidants and precursors to some crucial brain-supporting particles and neurotransmitters. Some of my preferred sources of anti-inflammatory, healthy fats consist of olive oil, coconut oil, avocados, grass-fed butter and wild-caught salmon. Eating good fats like olive oil supports healthy levels of cholesterol, which is an important element of appropriate hormonal agent synthesis.

5. Get Enough Sleep and Decrease Stress.

Sleep is also key to keeping our hormonal agents in check. A lack of sleep, long-lasting use of corticosteroids and persistent stress are 3 of the biggest contributors to high cortisol levels. A report published in the Indian Journal of Endocrinology and Metabolic process specifies that, Tension can lead to changes in the serum level of a lot of hormonal agents including glucocorticoids, catecholamine s, growth hormonal agent and prolactin.

Cortisol is a glucocorticoid hormone manufactured from cholesterol by enzymes. At the right levels, it's practical, but when you have too much it can cause issues. Since cortisol is regulated by the hypothalamus-pituitary-adrenal turning point and cortisol is the main hormone accountable for the tension reaction, keeping cortisol production at a healthy level through appropriate sleep and stress reduction is incredibly handy to the health of your hypothalamus (along with your pituitary and adrenal glands).

6. Workout Routinely.

Moderate exercise on a regular basis is exceptional for your hypothalamus along with your whole body. Certain research studies have previously found a gamma-amino-butyric acid shortage in the hypothalamus of hypertensive animal subjects. A study released in 2000 looked at the relationship between the hypothalamus, exercise and hypertension in animal subjects.

In this study, the researchers found that chronic exercise has a favorable impact on both gene expression and neuronal activity in the hypothalamus. Not remarkably, they also found that persistent exercise reduced high blood pressure levels in the hypertensive animals. It appears that exercise not only boosts heart health, but also enhances hypothalamus health, and improving both is very likely to help lower high blood pressure for people along with animals.

Studies have also found that there are a number of exercise-induced systems in the hypothalamus that may contribute healthy metabolic function in addition to energy balance.

Hypothalamus Disorders

Surgery, distressing brain injury, radiation and cancers are the most typical causes of hypothalamus malfunction. There are also some other possible roots of a hypothalamus condition, including:

Poor nutrition
Infections and swelling
Head injury
Bleeding
Eating conditions like anorexia and bulimia
Congenital diseases that cause bodily iron buildup

How can you know if you have something wrong with your hypothalamus? There are numerous signs depending on the source, but some of the most typical signs of unhealthy hypothalamus function include a slow heart rate, low body temperature, in addition to increased cravings and quick weight gain. Extreme thirst and frequent urination may also be indications of a hypothalamus issue as well as diabetes insipidus.

Some disorders that are related to hypothalamus malfunction consist of, but are not limited to:

Obesity

Multiple research studies have connected hypothalamus breakdown with obesity, a severe excess of body weight. This isn't surprising since we know that the hypothalamus plays a big role in metabolism and energy expenditure. The term hypothalamic obesity describes intractable weight gain after damage to the hypothalamus. Sadly, hypothalamic obesity can be a complication for some brain tumor survivors, specifically if they got their diagnoses as children. An approximated third of all craniopharyngioma survivors develop severe weight problems after medical diagnosis and treatment.

Adrenal Insufficiency

Low adrenal function or adrenal deficiency is associated with hypothalamus malfunction. The hypothalamus is part of the hypothalamus-pituitary-adrenal turning point and plays a significant part in adrenal insufficiency. Under ideal circumstances, the hypothalamus sends the pituitary gland launching hormonal agents to control sex hormonal agent production, thyroid and adrenal functions. The pituitary gland then has the job of communicating with the adrenal glands, sending it the stimulating hormone called adrenocorticotropin that's meant to prompt adrenal hormonal agent production.

Generally, the adrenals do their job, making correct levels of cortisol and other hormonal agents, and the pituitary gland and hypothalamus get the message but in people with adrenal insufficiency, all of the communication lines are thrown off. Low adrenal function signs may include lightheadedness or weakness.

Cluster Headaches

Recent research studies have revealed that the hypothalamus is stimulated during a cluster headache attack. A 2013 research study performed in China identified substantial boosts of functional connection to the right hypothalamus in cluster headache patients during intense spontaneous cluster headache in attack periods in contrast to those throughout the out of attack periods. Scientist concluded that cluster headache patients have a dysfunction of brain function connectivity, primarily in brain regions that relate to strong pain processing.

Other health issues related to hypothalamic dysfunction consist of:

Brain cancers
Hypothyroidism and Hashimoto's illness
Hypopituitarism
Gonadal shortage or secondary failure
Development hormonal agent deficiency
Secondary male hypogonadism

Hormone changes affect the hypothalamus, which manages body temperature level, and this results in the typical problem of hot flashes reported by ladies going through menopause. Also, if you'relady experiencing infertility, it might be as a result of polycystic ovarian syndrome, which relates to unhealthy hypothalamus function.

Precautions Concerning Hypothalamus Function

To determine if you have an issue with your hypothalamus function, your doctor will likely perform a physical exam and inquire about your signs. Blood or urine tests will also likely be performed to assess your hormonal agent levels.

If your physician determines that you have hormone deficiencies, hormone replacement medication will most likely be advised. Make certain to inform yourself about the side effects of any medication. Also, ensure to do what you can to naturally balance hormones.

Always use care when using vital oils, particularly if you have sensitive skin. Cease use if any negative responses occur. Always test initially in a little location right before using an oil all over the skin to make sure you don't have any allergy.

Why Do People Sweat?

Why is it that people sweat? You may know that it is a cooling mechanism for the body, but how does it work? This chapter will clarify how this cooling system works consisting of how to decrease extreme sweating and what to do if you are in a warm environment.

Sweating is when liquids (primarily water) consisting of minerals (such as salt) are excreted onto the skin. The majority of mammals sweat due to thermoregulatory reasons, so that the body's temperature is preserved, but it can also be used to bring in the opposite sweat due to the pheromones in the sweat. Sweating usually occurs in warm climates and during exercise, as this is when your body heats up and needs to be cooled down, but it can also occur when you are stressed out or anxious as a result of internal changes (hormones, hypertension). Mentally triggered perspiration is generally in particular parts like the hands and underarm, while physical causes (exercise, warm environment) are all over the body. Signals from the hypothalamus (the location in the brain that controls sweating) travel through the spinal cord and after that through the nerves where the sweat glands are promoted to produce sweat.

So how does sweating work? The boiling point of water is 100C meaning that it takes 100 degrees of heat energy to evaporate this water. Sweat develops a barrier against the external heat from the sun or other heat sources and our body, which leads to less heat energy being moved into our bodies - it is an effective barrier as the water and the minerals in the sweat need a ton of heat to vaporize. Sweating also helps to get rid of excess minerals, the other method of getting rid of excess minerals is through excretion. The real process of sweating reduces core temperature level, while evaporation of the water decreases surface area temperature level.

Whenever you are suffering in a warm environment or from a big amount of sweating you should always obtain lots of fluids and minerals - this is just one of your greatest priorities. Cooling your body down is another high priority, this can be done by utilizing cold water or ice, but there are other methods.

Hyperhidrosis is the right, scientific term for extreme sweating. This can be due to certain reasons such as genes, diet plan (spicy foods), stress, adolescence, anxiousness, endocrine problems, disease and warm environments. If you have had all of it of your life and members of your family have hyperhidrosis then the cause is probably genes - 60% of cases are. The main solution to hyperhidrosis is surgery, but there are other alternative methods just like creams, gels and pills.

Chapter 4: Help Your Brain Get in Better Shape

I'm certain that everyone has heard exercise, workout, workout to keep your body healthy. Well, you never ever hear anybody say workout your brain too. Your brain is just as crucial as the rest of your body. It is very common for people to experience a decrease in their psychological abilities as they age in age. It doesn't need to happen to you nevertheless, with a little effort you can stop your brain from aging no matter how old you are.

There are lots of ways in which the brain can support your brain. Workout, yes I said it, everybody says exercise to keep your body healthy, well it helps the brain too. But there are a lot more things you can do to keep your brain healthy. Sexual energy can even help your brain. It helps pass info between nerve cells. Decreasing your breathing rate can increase the activity of the hypothalamus and the pituitary glands. A really fun way to promote your brain is to try brand-new things. Walking back isn't brand-new but it sure does feel new and different there has been evidence that doing things in unusual patterns can make the brain bigger in size. Stimulate the senses too. Continuously keeping your eyes moving in your surrounding will keep the brain processing brand-new info and taking a minute to smell the roses or something you have not ever smelled before will enhance your brain.

More things you can do to keep your brain healthy are to get adequate sleep. Everyone really needs about 9 hours of sleep. The regular 6 to 8 hours does not cut it to keep a happy brain. Tension hormonal agents can actually kill your brain cells in your memory center. Even substances can worry the brain, caffeine; nicotine, drugs, and alcohol decrease the blood flow in the brain that trigger early aging of the body and your brain.

Thinking adversely can trigger damage to your brain too. When you feel sad or mad take a minute to believe is it truly worth sensation that why or am I over responding or being upset over absolutely nothing. Staying socially active and eat a balanced diet. These help too.

Certain foods can improve your brains' healthiness too. Things like fish, blueberries, nuts and green tea all assistance. Protein is necessary to enhance your psychological performance. Fish have protein and omega 3 that safeguard the brain and support its development. Blueberries are good anti-oxidants. They eliminate completely free extreme damage that triggers aging. Nuts and seeds are a lot like marvel foods for the brain, they have protein and fatty acids. They promote the pituitary glands and release growth hormonal agent. Broccoli, cauliflower, brussel sprouts, is essential for brain and memory health. Poultry, wheat, avocado, and milk will prevent age associated memory issues.

Green tea prevents Alzheimer's disease and has antioxidants that help prevent early brain aging. 2 cups a day will get your brain all the benefits that green tea needs to offer. Micro algae's including seaweed, kelp, spirulina, and chlorella are high energy supplements that help the over all brain function. There are other organic supplements and natural items that can help your brain. Option Health Supplements offers tons of natural items that will help your brain. There is focus supplements, memory supplements, in addition to other ones that will keep your brain in pointer top shape.

An Explanation of HGH and Its Impacts on the Body

What HGH is and exactly what it does are questions many individuals have. Just because of all of the claims surrounding HGH, there is also a ton of uncertainty surrounding HGH. When something promises to do way too much, it gets lumped in with "magic tonics" and "miracle pills". But there is sound, sensible science to HGH and the benefits that increasing HGH levels can have.

It is initially important to understand exactly what HGH is. HGH stands for human development hormone, which is a single chain polypeptide secreted in the pituitary gland. HGH controls cellular regeneration, which is the repair work and multiplication of body cells. This is obviously crucial for development and the repair work of damaged tissue. Cells can only last so long right before they must be changed by new body cells. The environment around us is harming to our bodies, the air we breathe, the water we drink, the sun and gravity all take their toll on body cells. Changing the harmed cells keeps the skin, heart, lungs and all other organs healthy and functioning properly.

HGH, as stated, is the hormonal agent which regulates this cellular regeneration. As we age, we produce less and less HGH. When we are children, we have extremely high levels of HGH because we are growing, and when we are in our 20s we have the highest levels of HGH we will experience in their adult years. Into our 30s, the amount of HGH we are producing lessen, and the damage from the surrounding environment starts to accumulate and compound very quickly. This is rather obvious in the wrinkling of skin and graying of hair, but also has a strong influence on the body immune system, energy levels and inner organ function. Increasing HGH levels to a healthier level will stimulate body cells to quicker reproduce so that this damage can be repaired. This is how HGH can effect so many areas of the body, because no location of the body does not need to constantly be creating brand-new cells (other than the brain, which sadly is the only part of the body which cannot create new cells).

For most of the time since the discovery of HGH, it was thought that the pituitary gland was gradually losing its capability to produce HGH. Just recently, though, it was shown that the pituitary of an elderly person was just as efficient in producing HGH as that of a child. The problem instead, lies with the hypothalamus which is the control center of the brain. For one reason or another, the hypothalamus losses its ability to read HGH levels and stops sending out the signal to produce and release HGH. The theory behind HGH supplements is based on this. HGH supplements actually do not consist of HGH, but rather promote the hypothalamus to send the signal to produce a lot more HGH. It is a much more secure alternative to manufactured HGH which, among other things, are possibly harmful and a highly managed substance.

The stimulation of the hypothalamus through this approach is showing guarantee in regions other than HGH production. The hypothalamus is responsible for keeping an eye on body function and adjusting the body to preserve ideal levels. This process is called homeostasis. It describes control of body temperature level, hydration, salt and sugar levels and much more. Without a correctly working hypothalamus the body doesn't always fall into the ideal levels and this can lead to every little thing from discomfort to serious health problem. For instance, when the external environment is cold, the hypothalamus diverts blood flow from the skin to maintain internal temperature, makes the skin strengthen to more effectively insulate and might make you shiver to produce heat through friction. If your body were not to do these things it would be much more difficult to maintain internal body temperature level; but this is just one example. Stimulating the hypothalamus will help it keep track of the condition of the body and react appropriately.

This is just an intro to HGH and the systems surrounding it. Particularly if you originate from a background in biology you might have found the book much to fundamental and simplified. There is much more to learn, and I encourage you to take an active method in investigating HGH, the hypothalamus and the pituitary gland. Hopefully however, this chapter can be the basis for some of your future research.

The Endocrine System: The Music of the Body

The endocrine system allows the body to preserve a state of balance or stability. It does so by triggering changes in the regular cellular functions, processes and rhythms so they operate in harmony. Music is the organized rhythmic harmonic noises that beings knowingly produce. They view it, appreciate it and respond to it. On the strength of these truths, the endocrine system is the music of the body. And the orchestra plays on.

The endocrine system is a symphony of glands and the hormones they produce and release into the blood stream. The orchestra is the amount overall of the activities of the endocrine system and the cells, tissues and organs it affects. And the orchestra plays on.

The theatre is the body - with its skeletal frame - and walls and roof of skin, muscle, sinews, and other connective tissue in between. The price of admission is birth. The efficiency is constant and non-stop - for the orchestra uses.

The players on instruments are the endocrine glands themselves. Their music is the hormones they secrete. The maestro of this biological orchestra is the hypothalamus of the brain. Its numerous receptors are the ears noticing the musical flow. Its a lot of transmitted electrical and hormone cues control the production and release of hormones by the glands much like the motions of the conductor direct the actions of the gamers on instruments. The hormones in turn stimulate responses by the cells, tissues, and organs just like music causes psychological reactions in its listeners. And the orchestra uses.

Endocrine glands also react to conditions within the body just like players on instruments react to conditions within the theatre. It may be applause, absence of it, lighting, temperature, etc. Positive conditions heighten the performance and negative conditions may moisten it. Likewise conditions in the body which disturb the body's balance cause changes in the secretion of hormones impacted by those conditions. Some examples are an abnormal blood sugar level, pregnancy, fluid deficiency, mineral imbalance, etc.

The audience of this symphony is the cells, tissues and organs of the body that react to the hormonal agents. The psychological responses of the audience are the changes in the physical functions and processes in response to the hormones. The ears of the audience which govern the discrimination and gratitude of the overtones and harmonics of the symphony are the receptors on the cells and tissues. For it is the stimulation of those receptors by the hormonal agents which stimulate natural reactions similar to the music of an orchestra provokes psychological responses in its listeners. And the orchestra uses.

The metaphor ends though with the awareness that we don't deliberately produce or manage the music of our continuously silent biological symphony. Neither do we consciously service it or preserve it. But yet, the orchestra plays on.

The Tiny Spot in Your Head That Makes You Fat

Its name is the Hypothalamus and is the size of an almond. It developed first with the lizards and controls sex, workout, thirst, appetite and high blood pressure. All your the majority of basic physical requirements regulate within this place. Feel an urge satisfied and the hypothalamus is at the heart of the conduct. Think of it as a primitive center of your brain determining much of what you do and prefer. In fact, your hypothalamus is also like an orchestral conductor invoking your emotions into action and, when it chooses, ordering them to disappear away.

Take cautious notice, for this is what actually determines your weight. When things work out, and you stay your ideal size, then be perfectly sure that the hypothalamus is performing its role as it should. Give it the credit, for your conscious mind just doesn't really need to stress - it's all instinctive. Gain weight and be similarly sure that something about the hypothalamus has come to misbehave. Then you need to have a hard time inside your conscious mind in an attempt to manage your food consumption.

There are two essential parts to the hypothalamus: the lateral hypothalamus and the ventral hypothalamus. Hurt or medically cut one and you become inordinately hungry-- forever and ever. Do the same to the other and you never prefer to food again. Medical science has know a lot about this for some decades. What it has not understood is exactly how all this works to maintain your weight at its correct level, or trigger you to put on weight when things go wrong. Researchers are now assembling this story piece-by-piece and it is remarkable.

It turns out that the hypothalamus is a lot like an extremely intricate computer receiving data from all types of places in the body. It is not just a Fat-O-Stat, as they once imagined it, but a most complicated program that pulls all types of information together. It is what understands how much fat you have and how much you eat. It determines how much you really need to eat to maintain an ideal weight and when you should eat it. Then it tells you when you should stop eating when you do. Clever stuff that is.

In addition to the bodily info about food and fat reserves it also needs to take into consideration-- in addition to control-- body temperature level and level of exercise. There is even some evidence that it even takes some psychological elements into account-- like tension caused by expecting a starvation. What is commonly called the famine-reflex more than likely resolve this mechanism.

There is one major ramification in all this. When you put on weight beyond what is natural this either happens in the head or arises by malfunctioning signaling to the head. The positive side of the is you have much more control over what happens in your brain than you most likely think. Even standard things like blood pressure and heart beat are available to mindful control though you might need to learn how to do this.

All this verifies that methods like weight reduction hypnosis and hypnotherapy can have a great impact over your weight. Either you change your mental process in regard to food and workout spontaneously (which a little minority of people do manage to achieve) or you really need to set out to intentionally change the way you believe and therefore behave in respect of food. Dieting by itself alters absolutely nothing at all. The problem is much in your head as your body.

Hypothalamic function can be affected by head injury, brain cancers, infection, surgical treatment, radiation and significant weight reduction. It can result in disorders of energy balance and thermoregulation, disorganized body rhythms, (sleeping disorders) and signs of pituitary deficiency as a result of loss of hypothalamic control. Pituitary deficiency (hypopituitarism) ultimately triggers a deficiency of hormones produced by the gonads, adrenal cortex and thyroid gland, as well as loss of development hormone.

Lack of anti-diuretic hormone production by the hypothalamus causes diabetes insipidus. In this condition the kidneys are not able to reabsorb water, which leads to extreme production of water down urine and huge quantities of drinking.

The hypothalamus is a pretty forgotten or unidentified gland for the majority of people, but it truly is an element of our anatomy that plays a major role in our health on a moment-to-moment basis. If the hypothalamus isn't working correctly, there are so many things that can fail.

Together, hypothalamus function and pituitary function control all procedures related to our total survival. Hopefully, having a much better comprehension of the hypothalamus will help you to see why encouraging the health of the gland can really go a long way to enhance your overall health and keep away from a lot of serious health problems that can be kept away from.

What Is a Neural Network really?

The most basic definition of a neural network, more properly described as an 'synthetic' neural network (ANN), is provided by the creator of one of the first neurocomputers, Dr. Robert Hecht-Nielsen. He defines a neural network as:

" ... a computing system made up of a number of easy, highly interconnected processing elements, which process info by their vibrant state reaction to external inputs.

ANNs are processing devices (algorithms or actual hardware) that are loosely modeled after the neuronal structure of the mammalian cortex but on much littler scales. A big ANN might have hundreds or countless processor systems, whereas a mammalian brain has billions of neurons with a corresponding boost in magnitude of their overall interaction and appearnt conduct. Although ANN researchers are typically not worried about whether their networks accurately look like natural systems, some have. For example, researchers have accurately simulated the function of the retina and modeled the eye rather well.

Although the mathematics included with neural networking is not an insignificant matter, a user can rather quickly gain at least an operational understanding of their structure and functions.

The Background of Neural Networks
Neural network simulations seem a recent development. However, this field was developed right before the arrival of computer systems, and has survived at least one major problem and some ages.
Many crucial advances have been enhanced by the usage of inexpensive computer emulations. Following an initial period of interest, the field made it through a period of disappointment and disrepute. Throughout this period when financing and professional support was minimal, crucial advances were made by relatively couple of scientists. These leaders had the ability to develop convincing technology which surpassed the limitations determined by Minsky and Papert. Minsky and Papert, published a book (in 1969) in which they summarized a general feeling of disappointment (against neural networks) among scientists, and was therefore accepted by the majority of without further analysis. Currently, the neural network field is enjoying a resurgence of interest and a corresponding boost in funding.

THE ESSENTIALS OF NEURAL NETWORKS
Neural networks are usually organized in layers. Layers are comprised of a number of interconnected 'nodes' which consist of an 'activation function'. Patterns exist to the network

via the 'input layer', which communicates to several 'hidden layers' where the real processing is done by means of a system of weighted 'connections'.

The majority of ANNs consist of some form of 'learning rule' which customizes the weights of the connections according to the input patterns that it is presented with. In a sense, ANNs learn by example as do their biological equivalents; a child learns to acknowledge pets from examples of pet dogs.

Although there are several kinds of learning rules used by neural networks, this presentation is concerned only with one; the delta rule. The delta rule is usually utilized by the most common class of ANNs called 'backpropagational neural networks' (BPNNs). Backpropagation is an abbreviation for the back propagation of mistake.

With the delta rule, as with other kinds of backpropagation, 'learning' is a supervised procedure that accompanies each cycle or 'epoch' (i.e. each time the network exists with a new input pattern) through a forward activation flow of outputs, and the backwards error propagation of weight changes. More simply, when a neural network is at first presented with a pattern it makes a random 'guess' as to what it may be. It then sees how far its answer was from the real one and makes a suitable change to its connection weights.

Backpropagation carries out a gradient descent within the solution's vector space to a 'international minimum' along the steepest vector of the error surface area. The global minimum is that theoretical solution with the most affordable possible mistake. The error surface itself is a hyperparaboloid but is rarely 'smooth' as is portrayed in the graphic below. Indeed, in many problems, the resolution space is quite irregular with numerous 'pits' and 'hills' which might trigger the network to settle in a 'regional minum' which is not the best general solution. How the delta rule finds the correct answer

Since the nature of the error space cannot be understood a prioi, neural network analysis typically requires a large number of individual runs to identify the best resolution. The majority of learning guidelines have built-in mathematical terms to assist in this procedure which control the 'speed' (Beta-coefficient) and the 'momentum' of the learning. The speed of learning is actually the rate of merging between the current resolution and the international minimum. Momentum helps the network to conquer obstacles (local minima) in the error surface and settle at or near the international minimum.

Once a neural network is 'trained' to a satisfactory level it may be used as an analytical tool on other data. To do this, the user no longer defines any training runs and instead permits the network to work in forward propagation mode only. New inputs are presented to the input pattern where they filter into and are processed by the middle layers as though training were occurring, though, at this point the output is maintained and no backpropagation happens. The output of a forward propagation run is the forecasted model for the data which can then be used for more analysis and analysis.

It is also possible to over-train a neural network, which means that the network has been trained exactly to respond to only one type of input; which is much like rote memorization. If this should happen then learning can no longer take place and the network is referred to as having actually been "grandmothered" in neural network lingo. In real-world applications this situation is not really useful since one would need a separate network for each new kind of input.

The Advantages
Neural networks, with their exceptional capability to derive meaning from complicated or inaccurate data, can be used to extract patterns and detect trends that are too complicated to be discovered by either people or other computer system techniques. A trained neural network can be thought of as an "professional" in the classification of information it has been offered to evaluate. This expert can then be used to supply projections given new circumstances of interest and respond to "what if" questions.

Other benefits consist of:
Adaptive learning: A capability to learn how to do jobs based upon the information given for training or preliminary experience.

Self-Organization: An ANN can develop its own company or representation of the information it gets throughout learning time.

Actual Time Operation: ANN computations might be performed in parallel, and special hardware gadgets are being created and produced which make the most of this ability.

Fault Tolerance through Redundant Information Coding: Partial destruction of a network results in the matching destruction of performance. Nevertheless, some network capabilities might be retained even with major network damage.

A neural network runs comparable to the brain's neural network. A nerve cell in a neural network is an easy mathematical function recording and organizing info according to architecture. The network carefully looks like analytical approaches like curve fitting and regression analysis.

Other advantages consist of:
Adaptive learning: An ability to learn how to do tasks based upon the data given for training or preliminary experience.

Self-Organization: An ANN can produce its own company or depiction of the information it gets throughout learning time.

Actual Time Operation: ANN calculations might be carried out in parallel, and special hardware gadgets are being created and produced which benefit from this ability.

Fault Tolerance through Redundant Information Coding: Partial damage of a network causes the corresponding deterioration of efficiency. However, some network abilities might be maintained even with major network damage.

How It Functions

A neural network runs comparable to the brain's neural network. A nerve cell in a neural network is an easy mathematical function capturing and organizing information according to architecture. The network carefully looks like statistical techniques just like curve fitting and regression analysis.

A neural network consists of layers of interconnected nodes. Each node is a perceptron and looks like a several direct regression. The perceptron feeds the signal created by a multiple direct regression into an activation function that may be nonlinear.

In a multi-layered perceptron (MLP), perceptrons are organized in interconnected layers. The input layer receives input patterns. The output layer contains categories or output signals to which input patterns might map. For example, the patterns may be a list of quantities for technical indicators regarding a security; prospective outputs could be purchase, hold or sell. Hidden layers adjust the weightings on the inputs till the error of the neural network is minimal. It is thought that covert layers extract prominent features in the input data that have predictive power with respect to the outputs. This defines feature extraction, which performs a function comparable to analytical methods like principal element analysis.

Applying the Neural Networks

Neural networks are extensively used in financial operations, enterprise preparation, trading, company analytics and item upkeep. Neural networks are very common in organisation applications just like forecasting and market research options, scams detection and threat evaluation.

A neural network analyzes price data and discovers chances for making trade decisions based upon completely examined data. The networks can identify subtle nonlinear interdependencies and patterns other techniques of technical analysis cannot discover. Nevertheless, a 10% boost in effectiveness is all an investor can expect from a neural network. There will always be data sets and job classes for which formerly used algorithms stay exceptional. The algorithm is not what matters; it is the well-prepared input information on the targeted sign that determines the success of a neural network.

How Are They Different from Traditional Computer Systems?

To better comprehend artificial neural computing it is very important to know first how a conventional 'serial' computer and its software process info. A serial computer has a central processing unit that can address a range of memory areas where data and instructions are stored. Calculations are made by the processor checking out a guideline in addition to any data the instruction requires from memory addresses, the direction is then carried out and the actual results are saved in a specified memory area as needed. In a serial system (and a basic parallel one as well) the computational steps are deterministic, consecutive and rational, and the state of an offered variable can be tracked from one operation to another.

In comparison, ANNs aren't sequential or necessarily deterministic. There are no complicated central processing units, rather there are lots of simple ones which usually not do anything more than take the weighted sum of their inputs from other processors. ANNs do not perform configured instructions; they respond in parallel (either simulated or real) to the pattern of inputs presented to it. There are also no separate memory addresses for storing data. Instead, info is contained in the overall activation 'state' of the network. 'Knowledge' is therefore represented by the network itself, which is rather literally more than the amount of its individual elements.

Which Applications Are They for?
Neural networks are universal approximators, and they work best if the system you are using them to model has a high tolerance to mistake. One would for that reason not be advised to use a neural network to balance one's cheque book. Nevertheless they work very well for:

Catching associations or discovering consistencies within a set of patterns;
Where the volume, number of variables or diversity of the data is very great;
The relationships between variables are slightly understood; or,
The relationships are hard to describe properly with standard techniques.

What Are the Limits?
There are tons of benefits and limitations to neural network analysis and to discuss this subject effectively we would have to take a look at each individual type of network, which isn't needed for this general discussion. In reference to backpropagational networks nevertheless, there are some particular problems prospective users should be aware of.

Backpropagational neural networks (and many other types of networks) are in a sense the supreme 'black boxes'. Apart from specifying the general architecture of a network and perhaps initially seeding it with a random numbers, the user has no other role than to feed it input and watch it train and wait for the output. In simple fact, it has been said that with backpropagation, "you practically don't know what you're doing". Some software application freely readily available software plans (NevProp, bp, Mactivation) do allow the user to sample the networks 'progress' at routine time intervals, but the learning itself advances by itself. The end product of the activity is a skilled network that provides no equations or coefficients specifying a relationship (as in regression) beyond its own internal mathematics. The network 'IS' the final formula of the relationship.

Backpropagational networks also tend to be slower to train than other kinds of networks and sometimes require thousands of dates. If operated on a really parallel computer system this issue is not really an issue, but if the BPNN is being simulated on standard serial device (i.e. a single SPARC, Mac or PC) training can take a while. This is since the machines CPU should calculate the function of each node and connection independently, which can be problematic in very large networks with a large amount of information. Nevertheless, the speed of most present machines is such that this is usually not much of a problem.

Using Them in Medical Diagnostics

Diagnostics of illnesses is broad and difficult location. Its task is to detect an illness that patient with the symptoms have. This process is extremely complex, as not all illness's signs are specific to only one disease and often the signs are overlapping. Errors brought on by human element are not unusual in this procedure. To get rid of human mistake, in contemporary medication, different technologies are used nowadays. Some of them are clinical choice support systems. These are interactive computer system programs that assist the medical professionals at diagnostic the client's illnesses. Using info about a client's condition in the mathematical model the probable diagnosis can be determined. These mathematical models are based upon statistical distributions, regression models and artificial intelligence. A synthetic neural network a part of expert system, with its capability to approximate any nonlinear transformation is a good tool for approximation and category problems.

Medical diagnostics using neural networks
The synthetic neural networks (ANNs) have unique advantages over analytical category approaches. The ANNs appropriate in cases, where standard category methods flop, just because of loud or insufficient information. Neural networks also benefit in multivariable category issues with a high correlation degree. The diagnosis of illnesses is a good example of such intricate category problems. By right application of synthetic neural networks in this area, to obtain the connection of symptoms and appropriate medical diagnosis, this reliance can be generalized.

Based upon this generalized model, we can then categorize input patterns representing different signs of illnesses. Nevertheless in the application process it is not needed to define algorithm, or otherwise identify the disease. The application needs only input patterns. The entire illnesses diagnostic process can be separated into training and diagnostic part. In general the training process starts with the choice of target diseases for which the category issue will be related to. After proper choice of illness, it is needed to figure out the specific specifications, symptoms and lab results which in detail define character of this illness.

The neural network is trained using this database and afterwards results obtained in this procedure are validated. If the results of the experienced neural network are correct, then the neural model can be used in medical practice. With this step the diagnostic process starts. The patient's data are processed by the neural network, which identifies the possible medical diagnosis. This result is then validated by the going to physician. The last medical diagnosis is result of physician's choice, who based on his own experiences, evaluates all aspects of the disease and the outcome of neural network classification.

Chapter 6: The Creation of Databases

In creating process of database for neural network training it is needed that this data define the scientific status of the client effectively. The data which represents unneeded or inaccurate information about the client's medical diagnosis should not be used. The selection process of suitable particular data is medical professional's task. Most often these data are basic information about the patient's health state, actual results of biochemical analyzes, signs and other info that helps determine the correct medical diagnosis. All these information of one patient which were gathered and assessed represent one input pattern of neural network.

The ability of generalization of the found reliance between symptoms and medical diagnosis heavily depends on the input patterns used in the training procedure. The database needs to therefore contain an adequate amount of reputable patterns which identify the medical diagnosis. This will make it possible for in the training process of the neural network to approximate the surprise reliance in the information set and to use this knowledge to generalize in client's diagnostic cases, even for cases which are not in the training data. The database structure has a form of table or matrix containing info about health status of patients and their diagnosis.

Forex Trading with Neural Networks

Today, we are seeing the increasing use of neural networks in monetary markets to help forecast prices with greater precision and the complexity and research is mind boggling. This article will look at using neural networks in monetary trading and their earnings potential.

The Human Brain V Computers
The human brain is just one of the most complex objects if not the most complicated thing understood to man. It is not just its remarkable processing speed and storage space that make it remarkable, but more importantly, its capability to learn and adapt.

Neural Networks Defined
Computer researchers have tried to write software that allows computer systems to simulate the learning power of the brain (computer systems already have superior storage and processing speed) and neural networks intend to help a computer system learn and adapt.

A neural network is essentially a system of programs and information structures that estimates the operation of the human brain. A neural network consists of a lot of processors running in parallel, each with its own sphere of knowledge and access to its own databank.

A neural network is "trained" by being given large amounts of data and a set of rules. A computer program can then tell the network how to respond in reaction to an external event and initiate reactions based upon the knowledge it has access to.

Therefore, in forex trading, neural networks can learn how to trade based upon the information fed to them.

Do They Work?
The answer is at present the human brain is and always will transcend, due to the simple fact it can BELIEVE individually. A computer can never attain the learning power of the human brain as it can only work with the guidelines it's set with.

A computer system program can trade, but do you need a neural network.
There are computer programs today, that don't use neural networks, that have guidelines that make money and neural networks don't have any benefit at all.

People believe that technology can fix every little thing, but the marketplaces are one location where basic systems can and do work best.

A Financial investment Simple fact
The fact is that 50 years ago 95% of forex dealers lost and today the exact same ratio applies. This is regardless of all the advances we have had in market research, computer systems and speed of information shipment. Keeps this point in mind if you want to win at forex trading:
Trading is an odds game and the application of science to anticipate is destined to failure.
There will never ever be a neural network with the power to learn and adjust like the human brain, as it needs to be configured by a human and there are limitless variables.

Keep it Simple for Success
If somebody tries to sell you a program or service based upon neural networking, request their real time performance history and see if you get one - chances are you won t.
People are always looking for science to help but in the markets forget neutral networks and play the chances.

Either with your brain or with a currency trading system, that's basic with just several guidelines - that's all you really need, do not look for more.

Integrating New Neurons

In the past, the field of Neuro research has a rigid belief that people cannot grow new neurons well into old age. But an impressive discovery in 1998 changed all of it. It's now believed that people can grow new neurons while they're aging. Now the focus of the studies primarily placed in discovering how these brand-new nerve cells integrate themselves with dignity into existing neural networks without triggering any potential problems. The research studies were performed in embryonic rodents and monkeys suggested that the neurotransmitter GABA, which usually prevents neurons from shooting, might instead be promoting new neurons to fire.

Amazed by this conclusion, a team at John Hopkins University focused to the part of the hippocampus, dentate gyrus. They penetrate a retrovirus into mice that makes dividing nerve cells fluoresce green. After that they can measure the responsiveness of these cells to different neurotransmitter.

Initially the neurons were sensitive to GABA that had diffused into the space between cells. After a week the new cells connected to established nerve cells, which transmitted GABA in pulses. In another week the cells formed connections to receive glutamate, the major stimulatory neurotransmitter in adult nerve cells. The results suggest that despite distinctions between embryos and adults, "freshly formed nerve cells must follow this series," says Yehezkel Ben-Ari, director of the Mediterranean Institute of Neurobiology in France, who is not connected to the Johns Hopkins work.

Apparently, an excess of chloride ions inside the young cells is responsible for their excitation by GABA-deficient neurons that the scientists engineered showed a two-week hold-up in developing connections and ultimately passed away. Johns Hopkins Neuroscientist Hongjun Song says the team wishes to evaluate whether applying GABA to stem cells at the correct time and dosage could help repair central nervous system injuries.

Stock Trading Made Easier

One such approach is in utilizing neural networking applications or commonly called expert system. This innovation has been created by developers which incorporate the old approaches and indicators together with new number crunching techniques to the marketplaces. Neural nets are advanced, trainable algorithms which reproduce particular major elements in the performance of the human brain. This supplies these items a distinct, self-training performance, the capability to formalize unclassified data and, much more importantly, the ability to make forecasts based upon the historical information they possess at their disposal.

Neural systems have been used increasingly in a variety of company applications, including forecasting and marketing research solutions. In some aspects, for example scams detection or maybe threat analysis, they are the indisputable leaders. The major fields where neural networks are finding use are monetary operations, enterprise preparation, trading, company analytics plus item maintenance. Neural networks is usually used proficiently by a ton of sellers, for that reason, if you are a trader and you haven't yet been introduced to neural networks, we'll take you through this process of technical analysis and show you how to apply the idea towards your trading method.

Many people have never ever become aware of neural networks and, if they aren't dealers, they probably do not really need to know what they are. What is really surprising, nevertheless, is the truth that a substantial number of those who could benefit highly from neural network systems have not even found out about it; accept it for only a complicated clinical idea or come up with it since a slick marketing trick. There are also those who pin their hopes on neural systems, lionizing the nets after some positive experience with them and considering them as being a silver-bullet method to fix any kind of problem.

Nevertheless, like any trading approach, neural nets are no quick-fix that will permit you to strike it wealthy just by clicking a crucial or 2. In fact, the correct grasp of neural networks and their purpose is important for its reliable application. As far as trading is concerned, neural networks actually are a new, unique method to technical analysis, planned for people who take a thinking technique to their business and are also happy to invest a long time and effort for making this approach advantage them. Most importantly, whenever used properly, neural networks has the ability to bring a good gain on a regular basis.

A lot of dealers make the miscalculation of following the easiest path - they rely greatly on and use the method for which their specific application offers the most user-friendly and automatic efficiency. This simplest approach is anticipating a cost several bars ahead and basing their trading intend on this forecast. Other traders anticipate price change or percentage of the price change. This approach hardly ever produces better results than forecasting market price directly. Both the simplistic approaches flop to expose and gainfully take advantage of a ton of the crucial longer-term interdependencies and, subsequently, the model quickly ends up being outdated generally since the global driving forces shift.

How Neural Networks Aid With Iris Recognition

There are variable ways of human confirmation throughout the world, as it is of high importance for all organizations, and different centers. Nowadays, the most essential ways of human verification are recognition through DNA, face, fingerprint, signature, speech, and iris.

Amongst all, among the current, trusted, and scientific approaches is iris acknowledgment which is practiced by some companies today, and its broad use in the future is of no doubt. Iris is a non identical organism made of vibrant muscles including robots with shaped lines. These lines are the primary causes of making everybody's iris is not similar. Even the irises of a pair of eyes of someone are completely different from one another. Even in the case of twins irises are completely different. Each iris is specialized by really narrow lines, rakes, and vessels in different people. The accuracy of recognition via iris is increased by utilizing increasingly more specifics. It has been proven that iris patterns are never ever changed nearly from the time the child is one years of age throughout all his life.

Over the past couple of years there has been significant interest in the development of neural network based pattern recognition systems, because of their ability to classify data. The type of neural network practiced by the researcher is the learning Vector Quantization which is a competitive network practical in the field of category of the patterns. The iris images prepared as a database is in the form of PNG (portable network graphics) pattern, on the other hand they must be preprocessed through which the limit of the iris is recognized and their features are extracted. For doing so, edge detection is done by the usage of canny approach. For more diverse and feature extraction of iris images DCT change is practiced.

Feature Extraction

For increasing the accuracy of our verification of iris system we should extract the functions so that they contain the primary products of the images for contrast and identification. The drawn out functions should be in a way that cause the least of flaw in the output of the system and in the ideal condition the output defect of the system should be no. The helpful features which should be extracted are acquired through edge detection in the primary step and the in next step we use DCT change.

Edge Detection

The primary step finds the iris external border, i.e. border between the iris and the sclera. This is done by carrying out edge detection on the gray scale iris image. In this work, the edges of the irises are detected using the "Canny technique" which finds edges by finding local optimums of the gradient. The gradient is calculated using the derivative of a Gaussian filter. The method uses 2 thresholds, to spot strong and weak edges, and consists of the weak edges in the output only if they are linked to strong edges. This approach is robust to additive sound, and able to detect "true" weak edges.

Although certain literature has considered the detection of ideal step edges, the edges gotten from natural images are generally not at all ideal step edges. Instead they are usually affected by one or several of these impacts: focal blur triggered by a limited depth-of-field and limited point spread function, penumbral blur caused by shadows created by light sources of non-zero radius, shading at a smooth thing edge, and local specularities or inter reflections in the vicinity of item edges.

Canny method

The Canny edge detection algorithm is known to a lot of as the optimal edge detector. Canny's intentions were to improve the a lot of edge detectors already out at the time he began his work. He was extremely effective in attaining his objective and his ideas and techniques can be found in his paper, "A Computational Approach to Edge Detection". In his paper, he followed a list of criteria to improve present techniques of edge detection. The very first and most obvious is low error rate. It is necessary that edges existing in images should not be really missed and that there be NO reactions to non-edges. The second requirement is that the edge points be well localized. Simply put, the distance between the edge pixels as found by the detector and the actual edge is to be at a minimum. A third requirement is to have only one reaction to a single edge. This was implemented since the first 2 were not substantial enough to totally get rid of the possibility of multiple reactions to an edge.

The Canny operator operates in a multi-stage procedure. First off the image is smoothed by Gaussian convolution. Then a basic 2-D initially acquired operator (rather like the Roberts Cross) is applied to the smoothed image to highlight areas of the image with important spatial derivatives. Edges trigger ridges in the gradient magnitude image. The algorithm then tracks along the top of these ridges and sets to absolutely no all pixels that aren't actually on the ridge top so as to give a thin line in the output, a procedure known as non-maximal suppression. The tracking process displays hysteresis controlled by 2 limits: T1 and T2, with T1 > T2. Tracking can only begin at a point on a ridge higher than T1. Tracking then continues in both directions out of that point until the height of the ridge falls below T2. This hysteresis helps to make sure that loud edges are not separated into multiple edge fragments.

Discrete Cosine Transform
Like any Fourier-related change, discrete cosine transforms (DCTs) reveal a function or a signal in regards to an amount of sinusoids with different frequencies and amplitudes. Like the discrete Fourier transforms (DFT), a DCT operates on a function at a limited number of discrete data points. The obvious difference between a DCT and a DFT is that the former an identified only cosine functions, while the latter a determined both cosines and sinusoids (in the form of complex exponentials). Nevertheless, this visible difference is merely an effect of a deeper difference: a DCT implies different boundary conditions than the DFT or other related changes.

The Fourier-related transforms that operate on a function over a limited domain, such as the DFT or DCT or a Fourier series, can be considered implicitly specifying an extension of that function outside the domain. That is, once you write a function f(x) as a sum of sinusoids, you can assess that amount at any x, even for x where the original f(x) was not specified. The DFT, like the Fourier series, indicates a routine extension of the original function. A DCT, like a cosine transform, implies an even extension of the initial function.

A discrete cosine transform (DCT) expresses a series of finitely many data points in terms of an amount of cosine functions oscillating at different frequencies. DCTs are very important to many applications in science and engineering, from poor compression of audio and images (where small high-frequency components can be disposed of), to spectral methods for the mathematical solution of partial differential formulas. Using cosine instead of sine functions is critical in these applications: for compression, it turns out that cosine functions are much more efficient (as explained right below, less are needed to approximate a normal signal), whereas for differential equations the cosines express a particular choice of boundary conditions.

In specific, a DCT is a Fourier-related transform comparable to the discrete Fourier transform (DFT), but using only real numbers. DCTs are comparable to DFTs of roughly twice the length, running on real information with even balance (since the Fourier transform of a very real and even function is real and even), where in some variations the input and output information are shifted by half a sample. There are eight basic DCT variants, of which four are pretty common.

The most common variation of discrete cosine transform is the type-II DCT, which is usually called simply "the DCT"; its inverse, the type-III DCT, is likewise often called just "the inverse DCT" or "the IDCT". Two associated changes are the discrete sine transforms (DST), which is comparable to a DFT of real and odd functions, and the customized discrete cosine transforms (MDCT), which is based on a DCT of overlapping data.

The DCT, and in specific the DCT-II, is typically used in signal and image processing, especially for lossy information compression, because it has a strong "energy compaction" property. Most of the signal information tends to be concentrated in a few low-frequency parts of the DCT.

Vector Quantization
In this work one Neural Network structure is used, which is learning Vector Quantization Neural Network. A brief overview of this network is given right below.

learning Vector Quantization
learning Vector Quantization (LVQ) is a monitored variation of vector quantization, comparable to Selforganising Maps (SOM) based upon work of Linde et al, Gray and Kohonen. It can be applied to pattern acknowledgment, multi-class classification and information compression tasks, e.g. speech acknowledgment, image processing or consumer category. As supervised method, LVQ uses known target output classifications for each input pattern of the form.

LVQ algorithms do not approximate thickness functions of class samples like Vector Quantization or Probabilistic Neural Networks do, but directly specify class boundaries based on prototypes, a nearest-neighbor rule and a winner-takes-it-all paradigm. The main idea is to cover the input space of samples with 'codebook vectors' (CVs), each representing an area identified with a class. A CV can be viewed as a prototype of a class member, localized in the centre of a class or decision area in the input space. A class can be represented by an arbitrarily number of CVs, but one CV represents one class only.

In terms of neural networks an LVQ is a feed forward net with one concealed layer of nerve cells, totally connected with the input layer. A CV can be viewed as a covert neuron ('Kohonen neuron') or a weight vector of the weights between all input neurons and the concerned Kohonen neuron respectively.

learning means modifying the weights in accordance with adapting rules and, for that reason, changing the position of a CV in the input space. Since class boundaries are built piecewise-linearly as sectors of the mid-planes between CVs of surrounding classes, the class boundaries are adjusted during the learning procedure. The tessellation induced by the set of CVs is ideal if all data within one cell undoubtedly belong to the same class. Classification after learning is based upon a provided sample's vicinity to the CVs: the classifier appoints the same class label to all samples that fall into the same tessellation - the label of the cell.

Chapter 7: Women's Brains

The male versus the female brain: is all of it in the mind?

The idea that biological distinctions in male and female brains trigger different behaviours, aptitudes and learning designs has just recently become strongly lodged in the general public brain, thanks to reams of research endorsed in ratings of popular science books. Male really do struggle with "man influenza" since their brains have more temperature receptors than women, so they feel more heat from the battle against bad bacteria. 'arallel" or sex-segregated learning is practiced from preparation till the start of year 10. It "allows you to do certain things that appeal more to one gender", says deputy primary Peter Buckingham, pointing out "a lot of evidence that gender relates to how people engage with learning and what kind of discovering they finest engage with". Yet the extent and effect of "necessary" brain-based differences in learning and abilities between the sexes is hotly objected to amongst scientists. Australia's many identified sociologist, boxing boys and girls into different learning styles on the basis of supposed natural distinctions is "educational nonsense" and "potentially harmful".

" Neurosexism".
The 2 least controversial biological differences between male and female brains are size (about 10 per cent larger in males typically) and a small structure within the hypothalamus (which is about twice as big, typically, in males). Great argues that, given the "daunting intricacy" of brain functioning, which depends on distributed neural networks and an excessive range of connections, synaptic functions and neurotransmitter systems, it is "remarkably ambitious" to try to relate subtle brain differences to psychological function. In the event for gendered difference in cognitive abilities, the test for psychological rotation efficiency includes demonstrating subjects a three-dimensional shape made up of cubes, together with 4 other comparable shapes. 2 of the four other shapes are the same as the target but have been rotated in three-dimensional space, and 2 are mirror images. When the job is to work out which two are the same as the target, about 75 per cent of people who score above average are male. This difference is said to be considerable in discussing guys' dominance in science, engineering and mathematics. Another proposal in assistance of gendered distinction is that high levels of foetal testosterone experienced by males in the womb completely "masculinises" the brain, leaving boys "innately" predisposed for normally male pursuits and interests. Fine points to "an unexpected number of gaps, presumptions, disparities and poor approaches" in clinical research studies of male-female brain differences. Her criticism of the infant face and mobile study has drawn her into a coruscating public exchange with Baron-Cohen, who implicates her of "extreme social determinism". Fine also asserts that the brain is not a "tidily isolated information processor", so test actual results are highly affected by social behaviour and attitudes, consisting of stereotypes, and can be quickly manipulated. For example, women have been found to do well also at mental rotation when they are told the white lie in advance that their sex is normally the exceptional entertainer. So why, if the proof is so thin, does the idea of a natural basis for distinction in male and female abilities persist? No rewards for guessing Fine's answer: "It helps to make the status quo seem fair, natural and inescapable. It's

reassuring to be able to take a look around at the significant sex inequality that still exists and blame different brains, rather than sexism, socialisation and discrimination."

Women's Brain Health Alert.

BRAIN HEALTH: Women's chances of developing Alzheimer's disease and dementia are DOUBLE that of a guy. Women have more than DOUBLE the chance of caring for a relative with cognitive disability. Present research studies show that women are most likely to development.
cognitive impairment quicker than men and not just because of age(1). The lasting impact this has on women is on different levels. First, more women are struggling with and dying of dementia. Second, since ladies are typically the caretakers, individual and monetary sacrifices are typically made that end up harming them. And finally, more women are leaving Alzheimer research work.
This ongoing tight spot for women in all parts of the world resulted in an International Alliance on Women's Brain Health. Their goal is to raise money for research, develop a clinical program, and organize medical professionals and scientists to encourage a quicker resolution to the problem. WomenAgainstAlzheimer's also joins ladies across the world to look for a treatment to Alzheimer's and is involved in the Worldwide Alliance. Right before this alliance, there were couple of organized efforts to.
fund research for gender-based studies or ladies' brain health. If you or somebody you know has been a caretaker of an older grownup, you know how demanding, isolating, and expensive this can be. It can keep you out of the labor force for years and harm your retirement. It can negatively change your relationship with your partner. This is in addition to the emotional toll it can handle you personally.

Marketing to the Female Brain.

The differences between ladies and guys aren't only well-documented, but frequently at the heart of jokes and good-natured ribbing. The fact is, males and females simply are wired differently. In human relationships, women tend to communicate more effectively than guys, concentrating on how to develop a solution that works for the group and talking through concerns. Guy tend to be more task-oriented, less talkative, and have a harder time understanding feelings that are not clearly verbalized. Guy typically prefer to peel away the extraneous detail and focus on the job at hand. To ladies, however, those specifics add richness and depth and are a very needed part of their decision-making procedure.

Here are some of the main neural reasons for these differences:
The Essentials. The male brain is organized in a nicely structured and compartmentalized way, where the female brain is more web-like and networked in structure.
Female brains have four times the number of connections between the left and right sides of the brain, which means they have to process info four times faster than men and take in 4 times as a lot of signals that must be filtered. Men have "The Huge T" - testosterone - which is responsible for lots of the male personality traits like self-assertiveness, competitiveness, risk-taking and thrill-seeking. Male also tap the right side of the brain, but not as usually as ladies, or

as deeply. While the male brain goes from point A to point B in a linear fashion, the female's brain runs in a more circuitous style.

The parts of the brain that manage speech and language are more pronounced in women. Yes, women talk more. Usually 12,000 words a day more. But that means, given the right scenarios, women are 10 -20 times most likely to share those great experiences and become walking supporters for a brand. Reaction to stress. Guy tend to have a "fight or flight" response to stress situations, while ladies approach these circumstances with a "tend or befriend" technique. The reason for these different responses to tension is rooted in hormonal agents. The hormonal agent oxytocin is released throughout stress in everyone. Nevertheless, estrogen tends to improve oxytocin, leading to relaxing and nurturing emotions whereas testosterone, which guys produce in high levels during stress, minimizes the effects of oxytocin. Feelings. Women generally have a larger deep limbic system, which promotes bonding and nesting instincts, and makes it possible for women to better reveal their feelings than men. The downside to this bigger deep limbic system is that it also opens ladies as much as anxiety, particularly during times of hormonal shifts like after giving birth or throughout woman's menstruation. One of the crucial ways in which marketers can better engage with ladies is to comprehend what makes her distinctively female. And understanding that doesn't mean they will alienate guys while doing so. On the contrary, while ladies expect more from the brand names and items they work with, guys ultimately benefit from those high expectations too. So if a brand name meets the requirements of the woman, generally it will exceed the needs of the man.

Do Women's Brains Really Make Them Safer Drivers?

Could the difference in the way ladies' brains work clarify why they have less roadway mishaps than guys or is it just a cultural distinction?

Women will generally take the role as childcarer meaning they are more likely to be in the home during the day. For that reason, they are less likely to be on the roadway throughout the most hazardous times, morning and evening rush hours, when most accidents happen. It is possible that when in the automobile they will be driving with children on board; this might make them more prone to drive carefully and knowingly. It also means that they're likely to drive less miles, providing less of an opportunity to be associated with a mishap.

Ladies are understood to be considerably better than men at moving concentration. Guys do more motorway driving while ladies tend to contend with the more difficult conditions in the area centres, typically having to handle children too so they are used to needing to move concentration and needing to respond quickly and properly. When driving on the freeway it is easy to fall into a lax mode, Motorway hypnosis is a well-known problem, you switch off making you slow to respond. So it's not much of a surprise that guys are susceptible to more accidents. Could the old argument that ladies are better at multitasking actually be true? If so, could this be another reason ladies tend to be more secure drivers?

Scientists really believe sex hormones could be the reason for the different driving capabilities between men and women. Women seem to be more knowledgeable about their surroundings, and also realize they are being asked to do something quicker than a man. The report goes on to show that ladies are quicker to change focus to deal with unforeseen events just like a vehicle taking out in front of them. Men nevertheless are supposed to be better at parking and map reading. This is likely to be down to testosterone, the male hormonal agent which aids space awareness.

How different are guys' and ladies' brains?

There are lots of studies that intend to check out the question of underlying distinctions between the brains of males and females. But the results seem to differ extremely, or the analyses provided to the main findings are in difference.

In existing research studies, researchers have taken a look at any physiological distinctions between the brains of women and men. They then studied patterns of activation in the brains of individuals of both sexes to see if males and females relate to the same external stimuli and cognitive or motor jobs in the exact same way.

Typically, there are no specific answers, and researchers tend to disagree on some of the most fundamental aspects - like whether there are any significant physiological distinctions between the brains of women and men.

Are there 'hardwired distinctions?'

Progressively, online articles and popular science books interest brand-new clinical research studies to provide fast and easy descriptions of "why guys are from Mars and ladies come from Venus," to paraphrase a widely known bestseller about heterosexual relationship management. One such example is a book from the Gurian Institute, which highlights that child girls and boys should be treated differently because of their underlying neural differences. Non-differentiated child-rearing, the authors suggest, may eventually be unhealthy.

Automobiles for boys, teddies for girls?

Some examples offered on these "innate differences" typically originated from research studies on different primates, like rhesus monkeys. One experiment offered male and female monkeys typically "girly" (" plush") or "boyish" (" wheeled") toys and observed which types of toys each would choose.

This team of researchers found that male rhesus monkeys appeared to naturally favor "wheeled" toys, whereas the females played primarily with "plush" toys.

Different brain activation patterns

Still, there are certain studies that determine different patterns of activation in the brains of men versus women given the exact same job, or exposed to the same stimuli.

Navigation

One such research study examined sex-specific brain activity in the setting of visuospatial navigation. The scientists used practical MRI (fMRI) to keep track of how men's and ladies' brains reacted to a maze job.

In their given activity, participants of both sexes needed to find their way out of a complex virtual labyrinth.

Another study found "rather robust differences" between resting brain activity in men and in women. When the brain is in a resting state, it means that it is not responding to any direct tasks - but that doesn't mean it isn't active.

Scanning a brain "at rest" is meant to reveal any activity that is "intrinsic" to that brain, and which happens spontaneously.

When looking at the distinctions between male and female brains "at rest," the scientists saw a "intricate pattern, recommending that several distinctions between males and women in conduct might have their sources in the activity of the resting brain."

What those differences in behaviour may amount to, however, is a matter of debate.

Chapter 8: Social Cues

An experiment targeting guys' and women's reaction to viewed hazard, for example, highlighted a better evaluation of danger on the part of women.

Vulnerability to brain disorders
A lot of scientists continue to point toward evidence that the distinct physiological patterns of male and female brains lead to a split up vulnerability to neurocognitive diseases, as well as other health-related issues.
One recent research study covered by MNT, for instance, suggests that microglia - which are specialized cells that belong to the brain's immune system - are more active in ladies, suggesting that ladies are more exposed to chronic real pain than guys.
Yet another analysis of brain scans for both sexes suggested that women show higher brain activity in more areas of the brain than men.
According to the researchers, this heightened activation - specifically of the prefrontal cortex and of the limbic areas, connected with impulse control and mood guideline - means that ladies are more vulnerable to state of mind disorders such as anxiety and stress and anxiety.

Brain activity higher in women than men, research study finds

Some brain disorders are a lot more typical in ladies than guys, but why? A new research study may help to shed light on this sex distinction, after finding that many brain regions are far more active in women.
Using a functional neuroimaging technique on more than 26,000 adults, scientists found that ladies have higher activity in numerous brain areas, consisting of those connected with impulse control, stress and anxiety, and mood.
When it concerns brain-related conditions, women and men are often disproportionately impacted. Foe example, according to the Alzheimer's Association, around 5.5 million people in the United States are coping with Alzheimer's illness. Of these individuals, around two thirds are women.
Studies have also found that ladies are practically two times as very likely as guys to develop anxiety over the course of a life time.
Tons of developmental disorders - just like autism and attention deficit hyperactivity disorder (ADHD) - nevertheless, are more typical in males. According to the Centers for Illness Control and Avoidance (CDC), autism is around 4.5 times more common in boys than girls.

Higher brain activity for women
The researchers came to their findings by examining brain scans from 119 healthy women and men, along with 26,683 men and women who had been diagnosed with a psychiatric condition, like ADHD, bipolar affective disorder, or schizophrenia.
Brain images for each individual were taken using single photon emission computed tomography (SPECT), a type of functional imaging strategy that gauges blood flow in particular brain areas, which is a good indicator of activity in that area.

The study exposed that women showed much higher brain activity in more brain regions than guys. For instance, at study baseline, their brain activity was increased in 65 brain areas, compared with only 9 brain regions for men. During the concentration task, ladies showed increased activity in 48 brain regions, while men showed increased activity in just 22 brain regions.

Women have more active brains than guys, according to science

women's brains are considerably more active in much more regions than guys s, according to new research.
The findings could help clarify why women are more susceptible to anxiety, anxiety, sleeping disorders and eating conditions.
The study by researchers from Amen Clinics in California is the largest brain imaging study to date. It compared over 46,000 brain scans from 9 centers and analyzed the distinctions between male and female brains.
Understanding these distinctions is crucial, the researchers say, because it helps to shed more light on how brain disorders affect women and men differently.
For instance, women are most likely to be identified with Alzheimer's illness, anxiety and anxiety conditions, while men have higher rates of attention deficit disorder (ADHD) and conduct-related disorders. This is a very crucial research study to help understand gender-based brain distinctions. The quantifiable differences we determined between males and females are very important for comprehending gender-based danger for brain disorders such as Alzheimer's illness. The researchers used brain scans from 119 healthy volunteers and 26,683 patients with a series of psychiatric conditions like brain injury, bipolar, mood conditions, schizophrenia and other psychotic conditions, and ADHD.
The research study subjects rested or performed cognitive jobs while researchers measured blood flow in their brains using single photon emission computed tomography (SPECT). The researchers examined an overall of 128 brain areas at standard (at the beginning of the research study) and during a concentration task. They found that women had greater blood flow in the prefrontal cortex compared to guys, which might help to explain why women tend to be stronger in the parts of empathy, instinct, partnership, self-discipline and showing suitable issue. It also revealed increased blood flow in limbic regions of the brains of ladies, which may also partially clarify why ladies are more prone to anxiety, depression, sleeping disorders, and eating conditions. Nevertheless, the human brain - regardless of gender - is changeable and notoriously challenging to understand.

Research study of Emotion: Ladies's Brains Are Wired for Compassion Almost everyone concurs that women, on the whole, are more compassionate than guys. In a 2008 Bench research poll, 80 percent of Americans expressed that view. Is this a sexist stereotype? Obviously not. Recently released brain-imaging research suggests that, in this case, standard knowledge is correct. It finds women's brains procedure compassion differently than guys s, obviously because of the distinctive way our particular neural systems progressed. Our actual results suggest that empathy systems progressed differentially in women, probably in connection with social skills consisting of maternal preverbal communication and psychological responses to powerless offspring, No gender distinctions were observed in the frequency of reported caring experiences, the researchers report. Nevertheless, what was going on in the individuals brain told a much different story. As the compassion-evoking photos were viewed, activity was observed in 2 parts of the brain the thalamus and the putamen, part of the basal ganglia in ladies but not in men.

Likewise, ladies showed a higher activation in the cerebellum, a structure governing detailed motion control that is also associated with judgment, selective attention and affective experiences, they report. The cerebellum may play a role in the decision to execute assisting actions.

The present findings suggest that women achieve the complex emotional-cognitive process defined as compassion through a more intricate brain processing than men by engaging prefrontal and cingulated cortices, The results agree with gender differences reporting a higher emotional sensitivity in women when viewing aversive and suffering circumstances.

So women: When the guys in your life seem insensitive to suffering, try not to respond with scorn. The issue, according to this study of emotion, is just one of brain circuitry. It shouldn't be hard to take pity on them; after all, you have a huge capacity for empathy.

Female arousal is far from an easy matter.

You might have known this already, yet now there's a scientific research study that proves just how complex lady's mind can be when it pertains to intimacy.

As it ends up, woman's brain is far more promoted than a guy's when they are excited.

A new book that just recently hit the marketplace announces that women are far better than men when it pertains to recalling the psychological times of their life.

" The Female Brain" women tend to bear in mind the psychological events of their lives better than men because women's brains are structured differently and include a much different set of chemicals than their male equivalents. The book mentioned scientific studies that used PET and MRI scans to support this conclusion. The authors also cited over 60 pages of referrals to support her findings.

In this regard, the book said that the primary difference between women and men is that ladies' brains had a bigger hippocampus, which is the organ in the brain that shops emotions and produces memory development. Women's brains tend to have larger parts for language than guys. The book said that these differences are more noticeable throughout the 8th week of pregnancy when the female brain experiences a testosterone rise.

On the other hand, and not surprisingly, men were found to have bigger brain areas for hostility and action. Brizendrine also exposed that guys' brains also have 2 1/2 times more space than ladies' brains for the sexual drive.

Here are some of the other intriguing revelations in the book:
Men experience love at first sight more easily than ladies, according to the chapter on "Love and Trust".

Ladies are more attracted to "in proportion" guys as such men are said to give them better and more frequent orgasm, according to the chapter on sex and mentioning the results of a research study including 86 sexually active 22 years of age couples.
Handsome and balanced men tend to be more unfaithful and cheat more regularly than men with "less well-balanced bodies."

On the last item, it appears that ladies now deal with a very tough choice: to either have a great sex life with a good-looking, balanced partner who will likely cheat on them or opt for a "less healthy" male who will be devoted but lousy in bed.

Leaders Understand.

BRAIN GAIN: When Science, the Guardian, Telegraph and Daily Mail all run a piece as they did in mid-November, saying in huge type that guys' and women's brains are not really different after all, it's really complicated for those who are certain they are, and as this column has been saying loud and clear.
A lot hinges on whether they are or not least the entire argument about distinction rather than equality being what is valuable in the executive market place.
Like so much in the modern-day reporting of neuroscience, it's much easier to opt for the appealing heading than the clinical truth. So in case Brain Gain should be considered espousing a view that the most recent science has now shown wrong, a little unpicking of the circumstance appears to be called for.

The influential study that men's and women's brains are very different in the methods they work came from the University of Pennsylvania at the end of 2013. Using a thousand brain scans of males and females, boys and girls, the composite connection scans that were extremely widely reported at the time gave remarkable visual proof of how different are the internal worlds of ladies and guys.
The company of male brains revealed very little connection between the two halves of the brain, with primary paths being arranged in a front-to-back manner either/or and linear, would be the easiest description of what was revealed.
Female brains on the other hand revealed a massive functional interconnectedness between the two hemispheres. Networked and inclusive describes the noticeable pattern well.
If one bears in mind that the left side of the brain deals primarily with what is understood, while the right side deals with the look for the unidentified, then there are some conclusions crucial to the full valuing of women in companies that can be drawn from these observations. They link carefully to typical observations about the distinctions between men and women but now have the virtue of a clinical basis for making theorized reasonings.
The very first such reasoning is that it looks as if guys may be particularly strong at analytical whilst ladies are resolution candidates. There's a big distinction between those two modes of operating. Ladies, it suggests, are not specifically interested by the finishing of something as they see that as only an on-going part of a solution constantly re-defined. Male, on the other hand, concentrate on analytical and outcome (obtaining a bargain of their identity from that

too, not to mention excuses for celebrating) but don't take the wider image so easily into account.

A second inference is that in not being so problem-focused ladies may appear (to guys) to lack focus. But the idea here is that they are scanning broader horizons. The person in the crow's nest of an eighteenth-century merchant ship might not have had a hand on the tiller but was the very first to find land, a potential friend or opponent sail, see pirates slipping out of a Barbary coast port, or give caution of what was out of sight from the poop deck where the captain's authority held sway. It might be that women are better tactical thinkers than companies normally give credence for.

A third reasoning is that no thought at all has been given to what organizational systems are needed to assist in the working of ladies' brains. This might become a major location for organizational development. If, as Laloux has suggested in Re-inventing Organizations, the future of quality in companies and their capability to keep skill will depend on the quality of relationships, trust and self-regulating regard, then it might be that ladies have a more user-friendly understanding of such procedures than is vouchsafed to guys. It's not that men can't actually learn them, but that they may be more spontaneously natural to ladies. We might be coming to the end of the area when, to progress in organizations, ladies have had to become the best guys they can be. All of these proposals could be put to empirical test. The future of management would then increasingly rely upon best realities instead of best guesses. The ramifications of these kinds of observations for management style also bear systematic consideration. And the list could go on and on. However, what if, as the reports initially pointed out at the start of the column, are right and there is no real difference between guys' and ladies' brains? That's where a vital take a look at the uncritical reporting comes in. What the reported study had been examining was nothing to do with the way male and female brains operate but whether there were some rather particular structural differences between them that could reliably predict which was a male or female brain. The researchers concluded that there were no such differences. The papers then said there are no distinctions between guys' and ladies' brains, but entirely left out the importance of the question regarding whether they operate in a different way.

It is of some academic interest regarding whether there are structural distinctions. But there are significant practical effects of the simple fact that there are functional distinctions. In countless homes this season guys might be the job supervisors, and need a great deal of praise for the way the tree was brought home and embellished so well; but most probably woman will be ensuring that every little thing comes together to make the festivities flow. It's different brains that do it. So guys are dying because they don't have ladies' brains? Program me the proof. It is the crossover moment. For the first time, more guys are passing away of prostate cancer than women are from breast cancer. Any GP surgery will provide a blood test to check a guy's prostate-specific antigen (PSA) suggesting cancer. All guys need to do is ask. The trouble is that, as all of us know, men are from Mars. They do not go to GPs, don't discuss health problem and believe in their own invincibility. Guy with their compartmentalised brains are naturally greater risk-takers and believe they will beat the odds. In any case, to yield the hazard of health problem is an acknowledgement of weakness very unmasculine. Empathising ladies from Venus, with their different brain structures that encourage talking and discussing problems, are more acutely familiar with the threats. One of the reasons death from breast cancer is decreasing is because women, better comprehending the threats, need action as an NHS priority and after that act upon what is offered. No parallel need is coming from guys. It is just another piece of proof that males and females are supposedly hardwired to think and behave differently and on this event men are the losers. Male's brains are more segmented, runs the argument, and their thinking is concentrated and focused in the right hemisphere of the brain given over to calculus and thinking. By contrast, the story continues, women's left and right brain hemispheres are more interconnected, with far more traffic in the cerebral cortex. These spaghetti brain structures are hardwired to connect the creative and psychological measurements of the brain with its logical thinking component, boosting women's linguistic and compassionate capabilities, helping them better comprehend people. They feel more, essential when supporting the young and shaping neighborhoods in the human evolutionary story. Male fundamentally are better at mathematics and building dams; women are intrinsically better at English and building houses. For each research study showing the hypothesis that ladies' brains are less compartmentalised than guys s, there is another knocking it down. There is no conclusive proof that there is more traffic in ladies' cortexes; no evidence that testosterone starts to separate out boys brain hemispheres in the womb; no proof that more highly compartmentalised brains enable more system thinking and no evidence that the resulting shorter brain circuits mean better brains. It is bunkum, from top to bottom, she argues, a kind of neurosexism. The greater truth is that we hardly comprehend what is going on in the brain. Instead, science is being infected by sexist stereotyping of men and women, triggering classifications and inferences to be invented that do not exist and validate ladies' continued subordination. For instance, evolutionary theory, which she does not contradict, is built on the truth of sexual choice developed by Darwin: the species has to be recreated and advanced by coupling between the two genders. That in turn means the winning of mates and achieving arousal by being appealing to one another. The nature of the attraction is intricate and evasive, but it does indicate fundamental gender behaviours that are different. Moreover, if male and female brains are as similar as Great suggests, how come autism is significantly more a male illness and the circulation of both genius and idiocy is more noticable in men than women? However, even the most difficult critics yield she is right to push back on the role of testosterone, its impact on brain function and the apparently deep neural differences between men and women. The science, they agree, does not back any of it. Checking out and listening to Fine, I would go farther the science is plentiful in neurosexism. Nor does choice theory challenge her position. It is flawlessly possible for men and women's brains to work identically with equivalent power perhaps men are not from Mars nor women from Venus, but from the same planet after all even while they behave in ways to draw in one another, as Darwin would forecast.

What is driving men's mortality rate from prostate cancer is not masculine brain structures it's the NHS costs half as much money on communication and treatment as it does for breast cancer. A century ago, researchers warned that winning the vote would put such neurological pressure on the challenged female brain there would be a 25% arise in female madness. Today, surely, we can see parallel statements for what they are: pernicious sexism. The Chinese saying is right: women and men hold up the sky similarly. It's time for everybody to act on that fundamental truth.

Science Explains Why women's Brains Work Better Than Men's Brains

New technologies have created a growing stack of evidence that there are inherent differences in how guys' and ladies' brains are wired and how they work.

We all know that men and women are two unique creatures behaviorally, emotionally and, yes, anatomically. These physiological differences reach the main apparatus behind all ideas and emotions: our lovely, uber-complex brain.

Our 3-pound tofu-like brain is what separates male and female habits, ideas, feelings, and feelings. Relatedly, studies show that in some methods the female brain surpasses that of us males.

New innovations have produced a growing stack of evidence that there are inherent differences in how guys' and ladies' brains are wired and how they work. ~ Stanford University School of Medication.

Hold the phones. We've got a substantial statement: The male and female brain are different. All of us know that males and females are 2 unique creatures behaviorally, emotionally and, yes, anatomically. These anatomical differences reach the central device behind all ideas and feelings: our stunning, uber-complex brain. Our 3-pound tofu-like brain is what separates male and female behaviors, ideas, feelings, and feelings. Relatedly, studies show that in some ways the female brain exceeds that of us males. (Yes, this author is a male so no biases here.).

In this book, we're going to go over the distinctions between the male and female brain, and how the female brain outshines that of man. Please remember that these observations are highly questionable. (As most things associated to gender-based distinctions cognitive or otherwise.).

Females brains regularly revealed more strongly collaborated activity between hemispheres. To put it simply, the female brain may be superior concerning how the left and right hemispheres of the brain communicate. Also called hemispheric lateralization, this inherent brain function has been shown in some studies to contribute in boosted cognitive ability. Additionally, in a comparable study, researchers found that ladies again, usually tend to have a higher amount of blood flow to the brain. Some studies show that a boost in cerebral blood flow (CBF) might impact cognition:

Using brain imaging information from 46,034 women and men, (researchers) found that women's brains were substantially more active (with higher blood flow) in much more regions than men's brains, specifically in the prefrontal cortex, which is included with focus and impulse control, and the psychological parts included with state of mind and anxiety.

Researchers presume that these differences in cerebral blood flow between males and females may help clarify why women tend to be stronger in compassion and instinct, along with self-control, while on the minus side why they might be more susceptible to anxiety and anxiety.

While there exist plenty of differences between the male and female brain, proactively looking after its health ought to be thought about a top priority.

With that in mind, here are some top suggestions according to professionals for keeping our most important property healthy:

Get mental stimulation: scientists have found that brainy activities promote brand-new connections between nerve cells and might even help the brain produce new cells.

Get moving: Exercise also spurs the development of new afferent neuron and increases the connections between brain cells (synapses).

Eat right: Great nutrition can help your mind in addition to your body fruits, vegetables, fish, nuts, unsaturated oils and plant sources of protein.

Enhance your blood pressure: Use way of life adjustment to keep your pressure as low as possible.

Mind your emotions: People who are restless, depressed, sleep-deprived, or tired tend to score improperly on cognitive function tests great mental health and relaxing sleep are certainly important goals.

Two Myths and 3 Truths About the Distinctions.

MISCONCEPTION 1 Women's brains are more balanced.

" It is really true that guys use one side of their brain to listen while women use both sides," says the Suite 101 (link is external) site with lost confidence.

This is a variation of the popular idea found in tons of books and sites that guys depend more than ladies on one hemisphere or the other for particular functions (particularly language), and associated to this, that women have a chunkier corpus callosum the bridge of nerve cells that links the 2 brain hemispheres.

One source of the myth is a theory proposed by the late US neurologist Norman Geschwind and his collaborators in the 1980s, that higher testosterone levels in the womb mean the left hemisphere of male children develops more gradually than women, and that it winds up more cramped. But the Geschwind claim is not true: John Gilmore and his group scanned the brains of 74 babies (link is external) and found no proof for smaller left hemispheres in male infants compared to women. Also unmasking the idea of greater lateralisation in male brains, a meta-analysis (link is external) by Iris Sommer and her associates of 14 studies, including 377 men and 442 ladies, found no evidence of distinctions in language lateralisation between the sexes. On the density of the corpus callosum, Mikkel Wallentin examined the evidence in a 2009 paper, consisting of post-mortem and brain imaging research studies. The alleged sex-related corpus callosum size difference is a misconception (link is external), he wrote.

TRUTH 1 Male's brains are bigger.

Men do have larger brains than women, even considering their bigger bodies. This has been recorded time and again. To take just one example, Sandra Witelson and her coworkers weighed the brains of 58 ladies and 42 guys post-mortem (link is external) and found the ladies' were 1248 grams typically, compared with 1378 grams for the men. Note, there's an overlap between the sexes, so some women will have bigger brains than some men. A Danish research study of 94 brains released in 1998 estimated that the larger male brain volume translated into a typical 16 percent greater amount of nerve cells in the neocortex of guys versus women.

TRUTH 2 There are sex differences in the size of individual brain structures.

The hippocampus, a structure involved in memory, is generally bigger in women; the amygdala, a structure associated with emotional processing, is bigger in men (link is external). It's also real that the cortical mantle (comprised of grey matter) is thicker in ladies, and that ladies tend to have a greater ratio of grey to white matter (link is external) (white matter being the sort of brain cells that are insulated). However, it's essential to note that these distinctions might have more to do with brain size than with sex in other words it could be that littler brains tend to have a higher ratio of grey matter, and it just happens that women tend to have littler brains.

MYTH 2 Sex-related brain differences explain behavioural distinctions between the sexes.
It's tempting to see the brain differences between the sexes, mythical or otherwise, and believe that they clarify behavioural differences; like guys' milk amnesia, their supremacy on psychological rotation (link is external) jobs or ladies' advantage with emotional processing (link is external). In fact, in many cases we simply don't know the implications of the sex-related brain distinctions. It's even possible that brain differences are accountable for behavioural similarities between the sexes. This is known as the payment theory and it could clarify why women and men's efficiency on different jobs is comparable even whilst they show different patterns of brain activity. Bearing this in mind, readers should treat with severe scepticism those evangelists who make use of presumed sex-related brain distinctions to support their claims about the requirement for gendered instructional practices.
It's also important to bear in mind that behavioural differences between the sexes are seldom as repaired as is usually made out in the media. Cultural expectations and pressures play a big part. For instance, telling women that their sex is inferior at mental rotation tends to provoke poor efficiency; giving them empowering information, by contrast, tends to nullify any sex distinctions. Connected to this, in nations that subscribe less highly to gender-stereotyped beliefs about ability, ladies tend to perform better at science (link is external). These kind of findings remind us that over-simplifying and over-generalising findings about gender distinctions threats setting up vicious self-fulfilling prophesies, so that males and females pertain to resemble unproven stereotypes.

FACT 3 Sex-related brain distinctions matter.
Whilst we should beware about how we analyze sex-related brain distinctions (Cordelia Fine reminds us (link is external) that the male brain is a lot like nothing worldwide even a female brain), it's crucial not to take political correctness too far and deny that distinctions do exist.

Seven Things That Make Males And Female VERY Different

We've all heard the phrase "Male are from Mars, Women are from Venus", but do you often feel like you and your love interest are galaxies apart, not just from different worlds?
Anyone who has dated just recently - or been involved in a relationship for any length of time-- can vouch for the fact that men and women believe in a different way.
Very in a different way ...
While it would be badly boring if both sexes were the exact same (think of how much you would miss out on making up after a battle.), often it would be useful to have an insight into your partner. Just how differently do we believe and feel?
While these are clearly generalities, here are seven fascinating differences between men and women that you may be able to relate to ...
-- Guys want to feel highly regarded. Women want to feel valued.

-- Women use approximately 7,000 words a day. Male use approximately 2,000.
-- When meeting lady, one of the first things that goes through a man's mind is what sort of sexual partner she would make. One of woman's very first thoughts is what kind of partner or provider he would make.
-- To guys, chocolate is just another snack. To lady, it's a food group.
-- A man's self worth is most closely tied to his earnings. Lady's self worth is most carefully connected to her capability to please other ones.
-- Male don't really need 3 different styles of black shoes.
-- To women, intimacy means nearness. To a man it means vulnerability.
In spite of these distinctions, men and women really want many of the exact same things out of a relationship. A dedicated, caring, joy-filled relationship is possible. After all, Venus and Mars aren't that far apart.

How they are Wired

Psychological tests have suggested for a long time, that men and women are each better at performing different kinds of psychological jobs. Guy stand out at spatial tasks, whereas women stand out when it comes to memory and instinct.
The research study concluded that this is because of the amount of neural connections between the left and right sides of the brain in women whereas neural connections in mens' brains were found within individual hemispheres. In other words, female brains are optimized for "interhemispheric communication" and male brains for "intrahemispheric communication." This difference in the wiring of the brain was found to happen during teenage years, at a time when other secondary sexual qualities develop as the product of sex hormones.

More proof

While measuring brain activity with magnetic resonance imaging during high blood pressure trials, UCLA scientists found that women and men had opposite reactions in the right front of the insular cortex, a part of the brain important to the experience of feelings, blood pressure control and self-awareness.
The insular cortex has 5 primary parts called gyri serving different roles. The scientists found that the blood pressure reaction in the front right gyrus revealed an opposite pattern in women and men, with men showing a higher right-sided activation in the area while the ladies revealed a lower response.
This is such a critical brain location and we hadn't expected to find such strong differences between men and women's brains. This region, the front-right insula, is involved with tension and keeping heart rate and blood pressure high. It's possible the ladies had already activated this area because of psychological tension, so that when they did the physical test in the research study, the brain area could not activate any more. However, it's also possible that this region is wired in a different way in males and females. We have always thought that the typical pattern was for this right-front insula area to activate more than other parts, during a task that raises high blood pressure, added Macey. However, since many earlier studies were in guys or male animals, it appears like this regular response was only in men. The healthy reaction in

ladies appears to be a lower right-sided activation. Distinctions in heart rate and blood brain flow throughout high blood pressure changes in males and females with obstructive sleep apnea and wanted to see if cardiovascular reactions in brain parts were different in healthy males and females.

Science Says People Aren't Really Wired In a different way.
There is no such thing as a male brain or a female brain, brand-new research finds. Instead, men and women's brains are an unpredictable mishmash of malelike and femalelike functions, the research study concludes. Even in brain areas previously thought to show distinctions based upon sex, variability is more typical than consistency.
Our research study demonstrates that though there are sex/gender distinctions in brain structure, brains do not fall into 2 classes, one normal of males and the other normal of women, nor are they lined up along a male brain female brain continuum,

3 sexist myths about the brain, unmasked.

From prospering in a guy's world, maybe it is now ladies who are wired for success? As innovation interferes with and levels the playing field, leaders really need to be mentally smart, able to manage contending needs and instinctive qualities more traditionally related to ladies. But is there any neuroscientific grounding behind these gender stereotypes? There are physical distinctions between a man and woman's brain in structure and chemicals, in addition to function. For instance, women and men's brains respond in a different way to stress and process psychological memories in a different way. However, these distinctions are simple to overstate and can distract from the larger messages that brain science has for everybody. We take a closer look at some:

1) Women are better at multi-tasking. This theory is based on the simple fact that the left and right sides of the cortex (the higher brain) are more densely connected in woman's brain than a guy s, implying that info can bridge the two hemispheres more effectively. On the other hand, men tend to have more front to back connections within a hemisphere.
We all struggle when we manage several tasks. But in reality, no human brain carries out very well when multi-tasking we end up doing each task less well than we would if we tackled it separately. In one study of 120 guys and 120 ladies, multitasking minimized efficiency by 77% in guys versus 66% in ladies. Consistent disruptions can also lead to increased stress and in some settings, like driving or flying or surgery, to serious security threats. It is better for us to move from multitasking altogether and focus on jobs completely and sequentially.

2) Ladies are less competitive and for that reason better at team effort. One of the underlying theories is that ladies are less competitive as a result of greater impacts of oestrogen and oxytocin (the bonding chemical) and less testosterone than the male brain. However, chemicals in the brain differ from individual to individual, as do levels of competitiveness.

3) Ladies are more mentally smart and better at using their intuition. One of the major differences between the male and female brain is in the orbitofrontal cortex and deep limbic

system. This system is involved in processing and expressing emotion, and has been kept in mind in some studies to be bigger in the adult female brain, resulting in the belief that women are better at articulating their own emotions and intuitively understanding other ones.

Again we should guard against stereotypes. Traits like compassion and compassion can differ widely with situation and under some situations, gender distinctions can disappear completely. Plainly, there are important distinctions in how each of us participates in critical leadership tasks, but gender is a poor clarification for them. The findings from brain science are nuanced and not necessarily deterministic and thus do not support simple explanations of gender stereotypes.

It is time for us to pass by neurosexism and develop a lifelong environment where both genders can flourish.

Chapter 9: The Triggers of Libido: Men vs. Women

Neuroscientists have much to teach us about the what's and why's of our sexual orientations. Merely on the basis of individual experience, you may be able to think some of their findings. Still, the actual results of their research on the nature and origins of our sensual interests aren't always intuitive. So there's a great chance that major spaces exist in your comprehension of where your sexual interests actually originate from. In simple fact, it's relatively very likely that some of your tastes, or tendencies, have puzzled you all along.

This specific segment of my multi-post coverage on the topic of human sexual desire will itself be divided into 2 parts. Here I ll be discussing the basics of male sexual predilections. In the next part I ll take up the rather different psycho-neurological hints that propel most women's sexual desire.

To begin with, it's vital to keep in mind that the literature specifically studying guys' arousal patterns (gay in addition to straight) has consistently highlighted their sensitivity to visual hints. As quickly as the lust-inspiring image signs up in their brain, they become turned-on not only physically but psychologically, too. Exposure to such sensual stimuli immediately activates the parts of their brain associated to getting an erection. And, as Ogas and Gaddam suggest, men's greater libido may be partly because of the fact that their sexual motivation pathways have more connections to the subcortical reward system than in ladies [or, in short] guys' brains are designed to objectify women. Annoyed ladies have frequently (and cynically) complained that guys' brains are located between their legs. But the authors more scientifically grounded viewpoint looks for to clarify the strategic and honestly, unwilled connection between the male's brain and his genital areas.

Men's and ladies' Brains Appear to Age in a Different Way

There's been a lot of badly thought-out stuff written about the distinctions between men's and women's brains and minds. In the absolute worst instances, sexist analysts use spurious neuroscience declares to offer proof for gender stereotypes men can't multitask as they use one brain hemisphere at a time while women use 2 (not true), or Louann Brizendine, author of The Female Brain, who says women are more emotional and understanding than men because they have more mirror nerve cells (ditto). But if you can get past all of this pseudoscience, there's some legitimately illuminating, serious medical research on sex-based brain distinctions some of which has crucial health implications. Consider one undeniable discovery in this location, which is that the sexes vary in their vulnerability to numerous neurological diseases. For example, Parkinson's disease (which hinders people's capability to move and causes tremblings) is more common in guys, and men tend to be diagnosed with the disease earlier than ladies; on the other hand, there's evidence that women are impacted more rapidly and adversely by the brain-cell loss that's associated with Alzheimer's illness. Research study into the differences between guys' and women's brains could help shine a helpful light on the physiological reasons underpinning these sex distinctions in illness vulnerability.

It's in that vein that a new brain-imaging study released in Brain Imaging and Conduct has made a small but essential contribution, by showing that subcortical (deep) structures in the brain appear to age quicker in men's brains than women s, possibly assisting to clarify why men are more prone to neurological illnesses that involve these structures, such as Parkinson s. The average age of the individuals was 32, with the youngest individual being 21 years of age and the oldest 58. Some of the most apparent gender distinctions they found are already well established in the literature: For instance, the men's brains were on typical bigger than the ladies' (a bigger brain doesn't necessarily produce a smarter brain; These become part of the brain involved in movement control and emotional processing, along with the thalamus, which is a lot like the brain's main relay station for passing info between different parts of the brain. After adjusting their data to represent the abovementioned total gender distinction in size, the scientists found several sex-based size differences in subcortical brain structures. For example, the women had more noodle in the left and right hippocampus (a structure associated with memory), while the men had a bigger caudate nucleus (involved in controlling voluntary motions) and larger thalamus. (Gray matter refers to brain tissue made up of neuronal cell bodies, as opposed to white matter, which consists of the insulated axons or tendrils via which brain cells communicate.).

Interestingly, the finding that the hippocampus tends to be larger in women has been reported a lot of times in the literature, yet it contradicts a recent research study that announced, after summarizing information from tons of prior investigations, that there is in simple fact no sex difference in this structure (prompting over-the-top pop-science headings like There is most likely no such thing as a male and female brain).

This just shows once again how complicated and inconsistent neuroscience can be, and how fast the media are to jump to extremes in the way they interpret this sort of research: One minute we're being told it's like the sexes are from different worlds, the next minute that there are no differences at all. The messy reality is very likely someplace in between. From a medical perspectives, the most crucial insight from the brand-new study involves sex-based changes in brain volume that correlated with participants age: For example, while both sexes revealed minimized overall brain volume and thalamus volume with age, only the men showed age-related reductions in caudate nucleus and putamen volume (the putamen is another subcortical area involved in movement control). Moreover, general gray matter (consisting of in subcortical areas) in the men's brains was found to decrease at a quicker rate than in ladies' brains which could be taken as a mark of faster brain aging in men. This study can't clarify why this brain-aging difference was observed, but the scientists hypothesize that age- and sex-related changes in hormonal agent levels might play a part, integrated with sex-related distinctions in how different brain structures react to these hormonal changes. Lots more research is needed to unpick these complex effects. The brand-new research study also can't say whether the more quick gray-matter loss in guys' subcortical structures is associated with their greater vulnerability to diseases such as Parkinson's disease, or perhaps to suicide (a recent paper linked self-destructive behavior with specific regions of decreased subcortical noodle), but this is absolutely a possibility worth examining.

What's clear is that we shouldn't sweep research on sex-based brain distinctions under the carpet in the interest of political accuracy, just because some misdirected authors use the field to make sweeping generalizations about men's and ladies' abilities and characters.

The brain capability of ladies, accounting for factors of sex mass to figure out that brain size was an unimportant factor in the determination of the relative intelligence of guys over ladies. Rather, even when considering only the little group of brain features that show the largest sex/gender differences, each brain is a special mosaic of features, some of which may be more typical in females compared with males, other ones may be more typical in males compared to women, and still other ones might prevail in both women and males. The question that appears is: do any of these differences impact the method which women and men perform the same jobs? And do such distinctions affect guys versus ladies' susceptibility to different brain disorders? Even if the evidence for natural brain differences between the sexes is undetermined, stereotypes are both consistent and powerful. Females have bigger brain areas related to intelligence.

In this regard, the book said that the primary difference between women and men is that women's brains had a larger hippocampus, which is the organ in the brain that stores feelings and produces memory development. Women's brains also have larger regions for language than guys. The book said that these differences are more pronounced throughout the eighth week of pregnancy when the female brain experiences a testosterone rise.

On the other hand, and not remarkably, guys were found to have larger brain parts for aggressiveness and action. Brizendrine also exposed that men's brains also have 2 1/2 times more space than women's brains for the sexual drive.

Here are some of the other intriguing discoveries in the book:

- Men experience love at very first sight more quickly than ladies, according to the chapter on "Love and Trust."

- Ladies are more brought in to "in proportion" guys because such men are said to give them better and more regular orgasm, according to the chapter on sex and mentioning the results of a research study involving 86 sexually active 22 years of age couples.

- Good-looking and symmetrical men tend to be more adulterous and cheat more regularly than guys with "less healthy bodies."

On the last product, it appears that women now deal with a tough choice: to either have a great sex life with a handsome, symmetrical partner who will likely cheat on them or opt for a "less healthy" male who will be loyal but poor in bed.

The Secret of Human Brain Size

A lot of times we typically confuse whether the brain's size has something to do with its capability. As all of us know now, the size of the average modern man's brain is littler than the forefather's, but our view of deep space (umweld) is much better compared to theirs. Does this mean that size has absolutely nothing to do with the brain's capability? Or there's something that we do not know yet about the mystery of human brain.

what about guys? Did the research study developed the same result? Right-handed guys revealed similar actual results for spoken abilities, but no correlation signed up amongst nourish-handed guys; for lefties and ambidextrous males, brain volume did not predict how well they had done on the language test. Witelson also found that for all men, overall brain size had no relation to visual-spatial abilities. Yet in on case, she found an exemption. In earlier work, Witelson had studied the anatomy of Albert Einstein's brain and revealed that though it was of average overall size, the inferior parietal lobes were broadened. These areas are crucial to processing visual imagery.

This study also revealed one intriguing findings As guys age from 25 to 80, the size of their brain normally reduces, yet age hardly alters brain size is ladies. And yet we still don't know the causes for this thing to happen. Maybe there are things that meant to be strange.

The Different Aging Rates in Guys' and Women's Brains

For several years, practically everyone has understood that males and females age in a different way. It has been common knowledge for some decades that men normally do not fare as well as ladies when it concerns growing older.

As a result, they're more likely to buckle down diseases later in life and they are also most likely to die at a younger age. Nevertheless, new research shows that the differences between women and men also exist in the brain. In fact, men and women's brains age at a far different rate. There are several crucial differences that should be explored more in-depth.

Perhaps the most important thing is that guys' brains tend to be better developed when it pertains to things like muscle coordination and movement. For example, they might be able to balance on one foot better or they may be more proficient at a particular sport.

They also may have better mastery and hand eye coordination than many ladies. With that being said, their brains also degrade at a much faster rate when it pertains to things like movement, balance and coordination. No matter how athletic a man may be in his prime, there is every chance that he will be far less capable as he gets older.

In addition, the part of the brain that processes emotions tends to age far more rapidly in guys than it does in ladies. What does this mean for someone in a realistic sense? It often means that guys are simply not efficient in handling emotions in the same way that they have always done. Even somebody who has always been extremely mature about his feelings and has managed to keep them in check during hard situations may find himself blowing up in rage or crying frantically for no obvious reason. This is not necessarily the fault of the person, but most likely because of the wear and tear within the brain.

As if that were insufficient, ladies' brains age more gradually when it concerns the part of the brain that is accountable for memory. This generally means that ladies can typically keep in mind better than guys as they get older. Practically all men have considerable wear and tear in the part of the brain that is responsible for memory that is straight associated with advancing age. This may even make them susceptible to dementia and other memory associated diseases.

One of the more intriguing possibilities is that way of life could be extremely responsible for these distinctions. Scientists do not yet know if the distinctions between males and females's brains is hardwired or if it is a direct outcome of the way of life that each supplier chooses. Without a doubt, a great deal more research will have to be carried out before any conclusive answers can be gotten concerning this specific question.

One thing is certain, there are a ton of differences between guys' and women's brains. As a result, more information can be found about these distinctions that can help people connect to each other in all aspects of their lives, particularly as they get older together. This research basically represents the tip of the iceberg and there is far more to be learned in the future.

Why Are Ladies So Hard to Understand? The 8 Huge Distinctions Between Guy's and Women's Brains

The majority of men always really believe that comprehending women is unrealistic. What guys actually need to understand is that we are absolutely different and, rather than quitting, we should try to embrace the distinctions and accept women for what they actually are, absolutely nothing like us. Only then we can use all of the knowledge to our advantage. The following article illustrates the differences between the sexes and explains how we can use these to our advantage.

Modern science has enabled us to study the male and female brains and come up with conclusions as to why we are so different. This is mainly down to how our brains are structured, and that's what this book is about. It will not teach you how to pick up women but it will show you why we are so different, and as quickly as you can get this around your head and accept ladies for what they actually are, then your it will become much easier to prosper with them.

Human Relationships: Women communicate much better than men, they focus on how to create a solution that works for the entire group, talking trough concerns, and utilizes non-verbal cues such as tone, feeling, and empathy. Guy on the other hand, tend to be more task-oriented, less talkative, and more isolated. Males have a tough time comprehending feelings that are not spoken, while ladies tend to intuit emotions and psychological hints. These differences plainly clarify why men and women sometimes have problem in communication and why men-to-men friendships look different from friendships among ladies.

What does this mean? If you ever spoke with lady, got deep into a subject and really felt like you spoke a totally different language well, this is the reason. In your step to comprehending ladies this is the first thing you really need to come down, THEY ARE very different. They are so different in simple fact that often we can't even communicate but, if you can be more in control of your emotions (and I know, no man wants to be in control of his emotions) they will not so much really believe that you comprehend them, but feel it. Now I'm not telling you to cry for hours after you watch "The Notebook" movie nevertheless, I am telling you that being in tune with your emotions results in you being able to communicate with her at a completely different level, a level that most guys do not get to.

Left brain vs. both hemispheres: Professionals have proven that men procedure better in the left hemisphere while women tend to process similarly well between the 2 hemispheres. This distinction plainly shows why men are more powerful with left-brain activities and technique analytical from a task-oriented perspectives while ladies normally resolve problems more creatively and are more familiar with feelings while interacting.

What does this mean? Well think of it for a second ... any problem that you had, you always hard about it this way: "I really need to get this done first, then this other thing, then this, and after that they all fit into spot and gets this done". Does that sound familiar? It ought to if you're a typical man. With ladies however, things are completely different and proves why men are better in some jobs (business, programming) and women in other ones (mentor, caretaking). This is another prime example that will get you closer to accepting just how different ladies' minds are.

Mathematical Abilities: An area in the brain called the inferior-parietal lobule (IPL) is normally considerably larger in guys, especially on the left side, than in women. This is the area responsible with mathematical ability, and probably clarifies why guys perform higher in mathematical tasks than do ladies. What's even more interesting is that this location of the brain that was unusually large in Einstein. The IPL also processes sensory info, and the larger right side in ladies enables them to concentrate on, "specific stimuli, just like child crying in the night".

Reaction to tension: In stress circumstance men have an action reaction that resembles "battle or flight" while ladies respond with a "tend and befriend" strategy. Psychologist Shelly E. Taylor first came up with the phrase "tend an befriend" after noticing that throughout times of stress women tend to take care of themselves and their kids (tending) and form strong group bonds (befriending). The reason behind these different responses to stress is down to hormonal agents. When someone is under tension the hormone oxytocin is released into the body. In guys, testosterone reduces the impacts of oxytocin as it is produced in high volumes during stress; this explains the reason for the "battle or flight" response. In women, estrogen magnifies the results of oxytocin leading to calming and nurturing feelings.

Language: The 2 sections in the brain which are accountable for language have been found to be considerably bigger in women than in guys, showing one reason ladies typically excel in language-based subjects and in language-associated thinking. It's also crucial to point out that guys generally process language in one hemisphere whilst ladies process it in both. This distinctions offers a little defense on case of a stroke, as women might have the ability to recover totally from a stroke affecting the language parts in the brain while guys might not have this same advantage.

What does this mean? Well it clearly means that women are better with languages than us guys, you need to have seen at least one lady that seems to pick up languages very quickly.

Emotions: The most obvious difference is probably the feelings. Women have a bigger deep limbic system than guys, it permits them o be more in touch with their emotions and better able to reveal themselves, which promotes bonding with other ones. This is one of the reasons that ladies function as caregivers for children. Regretfully this includes a downside as this bigger deep limbic system also opens women approximately anxiety, especially throughout times of hormonal shifts just like after childbirth or during woman's menstrual cycle.

What does this mean? Do you remember time when this girl you were talking with, was looking at the other girl, you saw, and believed that they were talking behind your back? Well they weren't talking, they just look at each other and communicate ... It impresses me in some cases how I have definitely not a single clue what's going on. Anyway this is most likely the most important difference and if understood can change the way you communicate with ladies.

Let's put it that way: women are in tune with their feelings - they are less in tune with their reasonable minds - so if you the man can make them feel great, all other things bare less importance. This is why when people tell you that looks do not matter you should actually believe them. Do not get me wrong, they do matter in some cases but, most of the time all of it bows down to how you make them feel. If you comprehend that making them feel great is what you should be doing (not impressing them with cash, looks, muscles or anything else) then you will have no trouble getting them into bed.

Brain Size: Normally, men's brains are 11-12% larger than ladies' brains. Unfortunately, this distinction in size has definitely nothing to do with intelligence, but does explain the distinction in size between males and females. Men need a bigger brain to manage their bigger bodies and muscles.

Discomfort: Men and women perceive pain in a different way. Studies have shown that ladies really need more morphine to reach the exact same level of real pain decrease. They have also revealed that female vocalize their pain and seek treatment much quicker than guys.

Throughout real pain, an area of the brain called the amygdala is activated. Research has revealed that in men the right amygdala (controls external functions) is triggered and in women the left amygdala (controls internal functions) is activated. This is the reason women appear to perceive real pain more intensely than guys.

So what can we draw from this book? Most importantly the simple fact that women and men are entirely different, but do you know the fun part? We can't live without one another.

What can we men do with this sort of info? Ladies like a man that understands them, although you can't understand precisely what she's thinking, you can still comprehend that she is different and the moment you accept her as that and respect her for it, she will see that you are different ... she will feel great about you, she will actually believe that "this guy comprehends me" not like the other guys ... and that is where your success starts.

Men Are Like Waffles

Why is it so hard to find out the opposite sex? Because our brains work differently.

Male's brains are actually proficient at focusing totally on just one thought and women's brains are truly proficient at thinking lots of thoughts at the same time. This difference can make it tough to determine what each other was thinking.

To highlight this, image a waffle. A waffle has many squares, each split by walls high enough to hold syrup. This is an example of a man's brain. Each waffle square is a thought or idea. In order for a guy to change from one idea to the next, he needs to get out of the square he is in and climb up over the wall to get into the next idea.

Now picture a plate of spaghetti. This is an example of lady's brain. Each spaghetti noodle is one thought or idea. However, each idea (noodle) is touching about 7 other thoughts (noodles) at the exact same time. Women are regularly thinking at least seven thoughts at the same time. Understanding how our brains work in a different way will help improve our communication with the opposite sex.

Guidance to Men: When she asks you to do a job, and then asks you to do 3 other tasks at the same time, remember that this is just how her brain works. Each thought is touching seven other ideas. Remind her that your brain works better when you can focus completely on one job at a time.

Advice to Women: Understanding how his brain is different should keep you from getting so mad at him when he is slow to change his attention from the television to you. Give him time to move into a brand-new waffle square when you really need him to change his focus or thoughts towards you.

Relationship Brain Chemistry - What to Do When a Female Cries

Tons of men are uncomfortable when lady weeps. Did you know that the chemistry of women's brains is different that a guy's? The chemistry distinctions come from our heritage of being hunters and collectors. Male's brain chemicals are built to help him in the hunt, while ladies' brain chemicals are built to assist her in event, nurturing children, and looking for assistance from other ones.

When a man is upset, his brain chemistry will push him towards being alone. This increases his testosterone, which helps him feel great. Testosterone also decreases his stress. When lady is upset, she searches for support, nurturing, caring and love. This gives her oxytocin, which helps her feel good. It also decreases her tension. Men's bodies long for testosterone, while ladies' bodies crave oxytocin.

Let Her Release Emotions

Bottom line, the resolution is for her to release the feeling through sobbing. This benefits lady. In women, weeping is a release of pent up feelings. The emotional centers of ladies' brains have 8 times more blood flow than a man's. Oxytocin tears are healing as they have chemicals in them that support healing and better feelings.

What To Do

1. Standard - overlook the tears. Don't let them bother you or affect you.
2. Intermediate - Listen to her. Enable her to emote with no resolution or repairing. The resolution is to let her cry. Have empathy and understanding.
3. Advanced - Touch her lovingly (and this means not sexually). You can do things like touch her hand, hold her hand or arm, hug her, hold her, or give her tissue and a glass of water.

Assistance Her, Don't Leave Her

Now a guy might want to leave her alone, which is good for a man. However this is not good for lady, unless it's to give her time to vent with her girlfriends. This may be good, but it also may be more harmful. It's very tough and painful for the woman to be left alone. When she feels hurt or sad, she wants comfort, nurturing and reassurance. All of these boost her oxytocin, which helps her feel better and decrease her tension.

If you really need to leave, it's finest to tell her, "I need some alone time. I love you and I'll be back." If you know where you're going and when you'll be back (particularly the latter), then it's really useful to tell her that.

In addition, the female begins to come up with all possible negative situations. Her brain is built this way. A lady's brain is actually wired to be the town alarm, to worry about all of the possible problems, and to seek help. The man's brain is wired to quickly examine the circumstance and do something if it's an arisency situation. If it's not an appearncy, the man's brain is wired to forget it. A female can't. So comprehending these distinctions in the brain chemistry can assist men to comprehend how to support lady when she cries. His benefit is a better woman.

Not Brain Surgical treatment

Everyone agrees that male and female brains are different, but it is difficult to tell just from looking how different they truly are. First, one should get past the obstacle of trying to find somebody ready to show your theirs if you show them yours. If you can, you'll note that the male and female brain are typically of around equivalent shapes and size, although the female brain does tend to hold in its stomach while being inspected and the male brain is often smeared with pizza sauce, generally sausage and green pepper.

But scientists have found lots of gender-related brain differences that are interesting even to those of us who aren't susceptible to spending our Saturday nights slicing gray matter with an Exacto knife and looking at it through a microscope since we do not date much. For instance, the sexes differ in the way we estimate time. Ladies approximate it fatter than it actually is, while guys approximate it much longer, specifically when in the room with other men.

There are also differences in the ability to envision things in three dimensions. Men's brains are better at this job, probably as women are too busy getting said things from the floor to have enough time to imagine them. Women's brains process language better, while men's process mechanical specifics, mathematics, science, and the music of bodily functions. These differences clarify why guys are better at piloting airplane, building bridges, and carrying out prop comedy while ladies are better at poetry and writing ransom notes to their ex-husbands when the child-support payments aren't on time. One exemption to the language rule is my next-door-neighbor Herman, who, with the right electrical voltage, can speak monosyllabically in thirteen languages, consisting of the African clicking language. But he avoid the last one as his dog recently attended clicker-training and will sit/stay for hours at a time.

One of the most current findings has been the discovery that ladies' brains can quickly handle several simultaneous tasks, while guys' brains, when confronted with needing to remember the names of their kids and store from a list, often huddle and roll around inside the skull gently weeping "Mommy." We know this from recent CAT scans of the brains of five hundred men who thought they were volunteering to taste-test a brand-new full-bodied beer.

Understanding how the brain differs according to gender might sooner or later help educators teach better, marketers target their markets better, and checking out aliens choose whom to abduct depending upon whether the laser thrusters are malfunctioning or the extraterrestrials really need their closets reorganized, their wardrobe made-over, and a new constitution written. We presume the aliens already know how to burp the alphabet.

How did the differences happen?

Why the distinction are there, looking at advancement (it's as men are produced for combating and searching and women for caring for infants and the social group). But then, how does the brain become what it should be in men/women? Is this difference present from birth or only in the future?

Certain hormones, we call them 'sex hormonal agents', begin affecting a certain person when it's still developing itself as a fetus. A male fetus, just 26 weeks old, shows a considerable distinction in brain from a female fetus. The disparities are found in the corpus callosum (bridge between left and right hemisphere), which in the brain of the female is much thicker than in the brain of the male. This is because of the fact that females use both their hemispheres, while males use mainly left.

Until the age of puberty, girls continue to outshine boys in making use of language and fine motor abilities. Kids show supremacy over girls when it comes to mathematics and geometry. These parts develop about 4 years earlier in boys than in girls. A recent study concluded that the brain of a 12-year-old-girl looks like that of an 8-year-old boy (when it comes to math). The specialities of the girls though, language and fine motor skills (such as handwriting), mature about 6 years previously.

Also, after adolescence, males consist of about 6.5 times more gray matter (' thinking matter') than women, while female brains contain about 9.5 times more white matter(' linking matter'). But a lot more appropriate is the simple fact that the frontal location and temporal area of the cortex are a lot more exactly organized in women (and bigger). As this explains the simple fact that girls typically call boys 'immature' or 'childish'. The lobes that 'make you grow' are much bigger, better organized, and earlier finished in women than in men.

Nature vs Nurture

But is it all nature? Nope. It all depends on how women and men use their special mental skills. Have you ever been just wondering 'why doe females always feel the need to gossip?'. As specified previously, women have a more advanced location for dealing with language. And therefore, they use it a lot. And by utilizing it, it becomes even more improved. So at the end it will be this 'substantial area'. If lady just does not speak very much because of her character or other circumstances, this location would not develop this much. And again, why this is can be explained by means of development or support in the first spot. Women used to have the job to look after children and establish relationships between social groups so they could stay alive. And we could also take a look at it as 'you got ta make do with what ya got'. For instance, when giving somebody directions, guys use a completely different part of the brain than women. Women use the cortex, and mostly count on landmark cues (' turn right at the supermarket'), while guys use a nucleus deep inside the brain, in the left hippocampus, and mostly rely on the spatial element (depth reckoning, 'go west here').

And then we have not even discussed emotions yet. Ladies are quicker and more accurate at determining feelings. Coming with that, is the capability to be more adept than guys at encoding facial differences and identifying change in vocal modulation (which clarifies why it appears as though every woman can sing exceptionally well).

However then there is a surprising twist when it comes to what practically everyone thinks 'women just have a lot more feelings than men'. This is not real. Ladies actually have a much greater control of aggressiveness and anger than men. Men just don't show their emotions, it's weak, and for that reason they always hide it, though their preliminary reaction to something is much heavier. Women on the other hand control their emotions and only show what is 'useful' or 'can't injure' but are also most of the time much softer in responding when somebody has done something very wrong.

What do we share?

A lot, actually. Almost everything. Not only is every brain different, and there are guys with a lot of emotional control, and women with more than average spatial-skills.

Take for example the spatial-skills. Every part of the brain can be enhanced, but how the spatial part? Well, by just walking through space. Doing sports. And boys get to do that much more than girls, which gives them a great benefit therefore. If we 'd treat girls and boys the exact same, they 'd eventually become the exact same is the theory. Which is quite sensible actually, and has research to prove it.

He Thinks, She Thinks - How Our Brains Are Different

Anyone with office experience knows men and women process info and communicate in a different way. Dealing with gender differences can prove difficult, specifically for managers and leaders.

Despite which market you remain in or the position you fill, male and female colleagues can experience a shared event and come away with different psychological stories.

We seem to be hardwired this way. Now that neuroscience is ending up being more sophisticated, with tools like brain imaging, what are we learning more about the gender divide?

Here are the key findings:
1. Feelings are useful. They make the brain take note.
2. Men and women process certain feelings in a different way.
3. These distinctions are a product of intricate interactions between nature and support.

Picture this: Several managers leave a stressful conference, where the conversation was dynamic and occasionally heated up.

A female manager jokingly asks her good friend if all men are missing a gene for level of sensitivity. A male associate overhears her remark and doesn't comprehend her reaction.

As he reaches his office, he silently shares a comment with a friend about female psychological reactivity and then alters the based on competitive bottom-line actual results.

Both are smart managers on their way up. But if you listen closely to their accounts of the conference, you would believe they had gone to different events.

Brain Distinctions
We can look to biology and the brain for explanations. In Brain Rules (Pear Press, 2008), molecular biologist John Medina points out these gender variations:

Males have only one X chromosome, while women have two. As it happens, the X chromosome is a cognitive "hot spot," carrying a large percentage of genes associated with brain development. The extra X in women serves as a backup, in case of requirement.

Men's and ladies' brains vary structurally and biochemically.

Guys have a larger amygdala, a structure that processes emotions. Their brains also more rapidly produce serotonin, a neurotransmitter that regulates state of mind, learning and memory, among other functions.

Ladies have bigger connectors in the corpus callosum, which connects the brain's right and left hemispheres.

Males and female react in a different way to intense stress.

Ladies trigger the left hemisphere's amygdala and keep in mind emotional details.

Men use the right amygdala and more quickly determine the gist of a circumstance.

What do these disparities mean in the workplace? How do they manifest in male/female interactions?

How the brain processes stress clarifies some of these discrepancies. As kept in mind previously, the amygdala governs many emotional responses, as well as our capability to remember them. After experiencing a terrible event, the female amygdala communicates with the left brain hemisphere. The opposite occurs in men: Their amygdala communicates with the right hemisphere.

As a result, women keep in mind the psychological details of an event, while guys remember the supreme result. Furthermore, women tend to use both hemispheres when speaking and processing spoken info, while men primarily use one.

"She's So Emotional ..."
The next time you hear men make the argument that ladies are more emotional, consider the following: Women have access to more psychological information. Their brains are built that way, enabling them to identify more emotional subtleties.

But too much emotional information can disrupt quick decision-making. Men can faster identify the overall circumstance.

Neither gender is right or very wrong, nor better or even worse. If we acknowledge the fundamental brain differences in males and females, we can be more tolerant and forgiving of each other's "shortcomings."

Why Men And Women Have Different Kinds Of Brains.

Apart from the physical and biological differences between males and females, current studies carried out by the National Academy of Sciences show that there are significant differences in the way human brain has progressed - not just socially and culturally, but also physically. From the findings, it would appear that women and men have brains with subtle differences, in the way in which the physical arrangement of the nerve cells and anxious tissues is concerned. While people tend to puzzle between the "mind" element and the "brain" element, it should be explained that when we discuss the "mind" aspect, we generally refer to the thought processes and the conscious, preconscious, and the unconscious states of the mind i.e. the manifestation of the physical brain. The brain, per se, is actually the physical structure of cells and tissues - the concrete part. The research studies carried out involving 1,000 young people aged between 18 to 22 years reveal that there could be a physical difference in the plan of nerve cells and structure of the brain between the two genders.

The differences in brain pattern.
Although physical development and sexual dimorphism slowly starts reducing once the individual completes adolescence, the minds might keep on developing, perhaps forever throughout the presence of the individual. As far as the brain is concerned, research studies suggest that the brain pattern in males more front-to-back oriented, while in case of women, it is more left-to-right oriented. Although the precise co-relation is not still completely clear, it would appear that the front-back orientation usually results into a specific functioning of the brain. Such a plan usually generates collaborated action and understanding. It would mean that the parts of brain accountable for these actions and characteristics are more highly developed than other ones. In case of women, the left-right orientation usually results into a higher

development of intuitive and emotional areas of the brain. This finding actually offers more credibility to the fact that women are more sensitive and mentally likely. It is not that they have these qualities owing to cultural reasons, but rather because their brains are more inclined to operate that way.

Gender roles and symptoms.
The dispute further continues as to did human brains actually progress to work in a different way in males and females over the centuries, or does cultural differences and gender roles completely dominate and make the brains as they are today. The research study still cannot actually prove that the evaluation occurred by itself, or whether it influenced the brain development in the first spot. The theory of evolution indicates what is used more tends to grow and develop more, and what is used less tends to become redundant with time. So did the brains develop in a way such that manly manifestation is actually different from that of womanly? There is no clear proof supporting or negating this fact.

Why It Is Very Important to Understand How Kids' Brains Are Different From Girls'.

verywhere - lack of experience and risk on the one side, care and steadiness on the other."
Men, when they turn out well are wonderful. But young males are so susceptible and so vulnerable to disaster.
More than half of university graduates in the U.S.A. are female. So much has been done for girls recently, but boys have been left behind. Problems emerge when parents and instructors do not comprehend the basic distinctions between boys and girls and for that reason flop to acknowledge what is actually happening in their boys' lives and what role they need to play.
It is that much easier for a mom to comprehend her daughter - after all she's a female and was once a little girl and daughter. However it is different for mothers and sons. Having a brother may help explain some things but it doesn't produce a complete grasp of what it is like to BE a kid - the marvel, the unlimited energy, the enjoyment, the vulnerabilities, the individuality and the testosterone rises.
The differences in boys and girls are hardwired. They are inherent and not socially built. Male brains affect how boys see, hear, feel, learn, play, connect, mingle, listen ... the list is endless. It for that reason has ramifications for how to teach, parent, encourage, understand and discipline boys.

Why guys brain is bigger than ladies?
hemispheric compartimentalization of function in male brains: the left side of a guy's brain is important for language while the right hemisphere is not; the right brain in men has a spatial function and the left brain is verbally orientated. Additionally, research shows that the proteins coded straight with the Y chromosome, that are so wealthy in lots of parts of the male brain, are entirely missing in female brain tissue. Females also have higher brain flow per gram of brain tissue than guys. In crucial areas of the brain, women have larger brain cells that receive more inputs than the equivalent areas of the male brain. And in lots of jobs, brain imaging research studies show that ladies used the most sophisticated location of the brain - the cortex - while guys perform the same job using less evolved areas like the amygdala and hippocampus.

When we speak about distinctions, we discuss just that. They are different - not better, not worse. The example of whether a spoon or a knife is better for eating your supper? Well, it depends what's for dinner. A spoon is better for eating soup whereas a knife is ineffective, and a knife is important for cutting steak while a spoon would be of no assistance. There is no difference in what boys and girls can do, but there is a big distinction in the best methods to teach them.

It is for that reason vital as parents and teachers to comprehend what male brains are good at so that we can enhance these talents. Its also key to comprehend their weak points so that we can save them from unnecessary struggle and find alternate methods for them to accomplish the best actual results, using a technique that works well for their male brains. To use the cutlery analogy again, there are many methods to give your child the right nutrients but if he only has a spoon do not make him struggle to eat a steak, give him minced meat.

Chapter 10: His and Her Brains at Work

Are guys' and women's brains different, when it pertains to the work environment? The answer is a resounding YES, and more importantly, science is finding that men and women work in a different way. When woman works like a man does, her health suffers.

Here are three things that are different in men's and women's brains:

1. Ladies Are So Psychological

Yes, ladies are more psychological than men, both on the positive and negative side. That's as women are designed to feel emotions for intensely than men. This also makes women more vulnerable to depression than men, which bears out in the data. Fortunately is, ladies can feel happier than men. But that doesn't mean guys are ruthless creatures. It just means that ladies have a bit wider variety of emotions than men.

On a related note, ladies have more electrical wiring available to detect facial expressions than guys. So women, you might have to give your man some extra clues to let him know if you are suffering and really need his assistance. Men simply don't have the wiring to know when you might be miserable till the tears start streaming. Then they get it. The bright side is, men can learn to detect facial expressions. Jobs like the cops, investigators, attorneys, judges, ministers, and poker gamers all require remarkable people-reading abilities, and men who do not have these skills can go through special training to select them up.

2. Honey, I Do Not Required to Ask for Directions

Typically speaking, men and women browse differently. Guys take more of a bird's- eye view to get somewhere, depending on an allocentric technique. Women depend on local landmarks and how they relate to their own physical location to get from point A to point B, taking an egocentric technique.

On an associated note, men also perform better on a task called spatial rotation. It was on our IQ tests in school, and it involved having the ability to mentally change the perspectives of a 3D object in our minds and recognize what it would appear like when it was turned.

3. Darling, You Barely Said a Thing All Night

Women have it all over guys in the spoken department. The brain is functionally organized and there are 2 parts on the left side of our brains (sometimes the right if you are left-handed) that manage our speech and language processing. Women's are bigger. Ladies are also able to bear in mind things better when the thing they are attempting to keep in mind can be connected with words.

Please keep in mind, these are all generalizations, so there will be individual differences that defy the averages.

Males and female at Work

Because of these brain distinctions, men and women's distinctions should be honored and celebrated in the office. Women who try to be successful at company using men's techniques will likely have health issue. One example is in sales: men tend to "conquer" or "capture" the prospect to close the sale. It's kind of like searching. If men have worry or stress on the job, they simply require their way through it. They can do this, being testosterone-laden. Women can't.

Ladies need to build relationships. They really need to embrace their worries and be supported, not fight their way through things. If they combat, they will burn out their adrenals eventually, or they will get sick often.

When we can honor the differences of each gender, we can also leverage the special strengths males and females take to the office, without trying to suit one another's mold. It's the distinctions that make it much more fun anyhow.

Gender Brain Chemistry - One Task Man Vs Multitasking Lady

Have you ever saw that a guy seems to focus only on the job at hand, whereas the woman's mind has so much going on all at once? Women appear to multitask with a lot more ease. Men are better at concentrating on the job at hand and finishing the job, before proceeding to the next one. Let's make it simple to understand why this gender brain difference occurs. I am going to clarify the differences in both gender's brain connection, and how that affects the way that they are able to job manage.

Gender Brain Connectivity

Women's brains have a bigger amount of nerves that connect the left and right hemispheres of the brain, and this makes her more capable of multitasking. Her brain is hard wired to talk, believe, listen, feel, strategy and keep in mind all at once. A guy's brain has 25% less connectivity in the corpus collosum, the link which supplies cross-talk between the two hemispheres. This makes his brain more able to focus on a certain task, shutting out all of life's other interruptions.

The One-Task Man

With less connection between brain hemispheres, he is less inclined to talk, feel and have the ability to articulate both at the exact same time. A guy will most likely focus on the job at hand, sometimes even ignoring everything else. Men separate their emotions and thoughts into different places in the brain.

For example, a man likes his partner very much. That is his feeling. But his job is to find a job to provide for his family. So his focus is job hunt, resumes, classifieds and networking. Then he forgets his marriage partner needs attention, love and to feel emotionally supported too. It is not that he does not really love her. It isn't that he doesn't want to listen about her day, but his brain is tough wired to focus on the task at hand and that is to find that job.

The Multitasking Female

Lady's connectivity is like an incredibly huge multi-directional highway that is busily buzzing along. Having more connectivity between the two hemispheres allows her to believe, do and feel feelings and connect to them far more easily. She is able to articulate her ideas a lot more rapidly. She also can have many ideas processing at one time. This is usually why ladies feel a lot more overloaded than most guys. And why he typically thinks she is just blowing things out of proportion.

For instance, lady wants to speak about the stress of her day. As she gets into about the 3rd or 4th thing, her spouse is ready to disrupt to use his way to solve the problem. This is the difference in gender hard circuitry for the brain. She is just seeking to speak about things and discuss them, which helps her focus and actually solve problems by talking them through. He is hard wired to fix them quickly and carry on. His brain is not thinking as lots of ideas as hers and, she can't help but to be thinking, sensation, talking, preparation, helping, and listening all at once.

How to Improve Your Brain

Aging isn't something anyone can stay away from, but there is an increasing body of research demonstrating us that there are things you can do, today, to help keep your mind sharp and your body healthy as you grow older. But how to improve your brain?

The latest bit of proof on vitamins, D in this case, and health comes from a population based study of over 3,100 European men (aged 40-79) that found the subjects with high vitamin D levels did better on both memory and info processing tests than subjects with lower levels.

Whether this important, though under valued nutrient protects the brain cells themselves or essential signaling pathways within the brain isn't clear, but the effect is certainly quantifiable.

The study, a joint effort between University of Manchester experts and associates from other European centers, appears in the Journal of Neurology, Neurosurgery and Psychiatry.

This latest work follows research that made news this past January recommending high levels of vitamin D can help stop the mental decrease of the aging brain.

Samples of blood were taken to measure vitamin D levels. Assessments also included how physically active the guys were, how they operated in every day life and reports on mood or depression.

In the end, the men with highest vitamin D levels did best on the tests and their cognitive efficiency was regularly better than those with the most affordable levels.

One surprise was that the distinction appeared most noticeably in subjects over 60 years of age.

Why might this be?

The scientists aren't sure, but suggest the vitamin may activate an increase in protective hormonal agents in the brain, however at present only animal research studies back this notion

Other evidence suggests that vitamin D may work to cool down an over active body immune system or maybe improve levels of anti-oxidants that work to cleanse the brain.

So while specialists can't clarify precisely how vitamin D works, they remain confident that it does undoubtedly have an effect on age related cognitive function.

As a fat-soluble nutrient, vitamin D is found naturally in just a few foods such as oily fish (salmon, tuna and mackerel), beef liver, fish liver oils, cheese and eggs. Prepared foods are also readily available, foods like milk, prepared to eat cereals, some brand names of orange juice, yogurt, margarine and fruit juices.

Even so, eating a diet with enough of this nutrient isn't as easy as you may think, and is the reason supplements have become so well-known. You'll want to speak to your own physician, to discuss your distinct circumstance, right before you start taking any supplement.

At present, the recommended consumption of vitamin D is 400-600 IU a day for those aged over 51, though at least 1000 IU per day is considered by a lot of to be a better suited level for older adults.

And while sunshine is also a natural source of the essential vitamin, as we age, our skin is less able to take in vitamin D from the sun, so older people depend more on food sources (or supplements) for this crucial nutrient. What's more, sun blocks of SPF 15 or higher, popular in our battle against skin cancer, are understood to block nearly all vitamin D synthesis by the skin. Being overweight or obese also makes your body less able to make vitamin D while you're out in the sun.

Estimates of vitamin D deficiency suggest that 50% of adults and kids in the United States aren't getting enough.

And seeing that vitamin D is progressively being connected to health advantages beyond the brain, things like minimizing arthritis, osteoporotic fractures, not to point out heart disease and even some cancers, there's never been a better time to make sure you're getting enough.

some considerable distinctions

Do the physiological distinctions between women and men sex organs, facial hair, and so forth reach our brains? The question has been as difficult to address as it has been controversial. Now, the largest brain-imaging study of its kind certainly finds some sex-specific patterns, but in general more similarities than differences. The work raises new questions about how brain differences between the sexes might affect intelligence and behavior.

For decades, brain researchers have observed that typically, male brains tend to have a little higher total brain volume than female ones, even when corrected for males bigger typical body size. But it has shown notoriously difficult to pin down precisely which foundations within the brain are more or less large. The majority of studies have looked at relatively small sample sizes typically fewer than 100 brains making large-scale conclusions unrealistic.

Adjusting for age, usually, they found that ladies tended to have significantly thicker cortices than guys. Thicker cortices have been connected with higher scores on a variety of cognitive and general intelligence tests. Meanwhile, guys had higher brain volumes than women in every subcortical region they looked at, consisting of the hippocampus (which plays broad roles in memory and spatial awareness), the amygdala (feelings, memory, and decision-making), striatum (learning, inhibition, and reward-processing), and thalamus (processing and passing on sensory information to other parts of the brain).

When the scientists changed the numbers to look at the subcortical regions relative to overall brain size, the contrasts became much closer: There were only 14 areas where guys had higher brain volume and 10 regions where ladies did.

Volumes and cortical thickness between men also tended to differ much more than they did between ladies, the researchers report this month in a paper posted to the bioRxiv server, and that makes short articles available right before they have been peer examined.

That's intriguing since it lines up with former work taking a look at sex and IQ tests. [That former research study] finds no typical distinction in intelligence, but males were more variable than women, Ritchie says. This is why our finding that male participants brains were, in most steps, more variable than female individuals brains is so fascinating. It fits with a ton of other evidence that appears to point towards males being more variable physically and mentally.

Despite the study's constant sex-linked patterns, the researchers also found substantial overlap between males and females in brain volume and cortical thickness, just as you may find in height. To put it simply, just by taking a look at the brain scan, or height, of somebody plucked at random from the study, scientists would be hard pushed to say whether it came from a man or lady. That suggests both sexes brains are far more comparable than they are different.

The research study didn't account for whether individuals gender matched their natural designation as male or female.

A new study on the physical makeup of the human brain has shown that women and men have differently formed brains, with ladies having thicker cortices a function typically connected with intelligence and men having bigger brains overall.

Through usage of MRI machines, researchers found that ladies' brains had bigger subregions of the cortex a part of the brain associated with memory, sensory input, learning, and making choices. Females's brains also tended to look more comparable to each aside from men's brains, which on the entire revealed greater variety in size and shape.

While general structural differences between men and women's brains do appear to exist, they stay minor sufficient to make it impossible to differentiate an individual's gender exclusively by taking a look at a brain. Researchers have hypothesized that these differences in brain structure may account for gender-specific abilities and/or conduct distinctions between the sexes, but Ritchie said that the research study was all about describing the distinctions instead of the causes.

The differences in males and females even reach the way our brains are built.

In the largest study yet on sex differences in the physical makeup of the human brain, scientists from the University of Edinburgh in Scotland have revealed that women and men do, in fact, have different brain structures and sizes. Ladies tend to have thicker cortices, which are connected with intelligence, whereas guys' brains tend to be larger general. Although these distinctions can't prove that women and men behave in a different way, they could shed light on why some medications work better in men better than women, and vice versa.

Scientist looked at the brains of over 5,200 participants older than 40, approximately half guys and half ladies. This group became part of the bigger UK Biobank research study, which is in the middle of gathering health information on over 500,000 people. For this particular study, patients set in a structural magnetic resonance imaging. These MRIs are able to parse out different kinds of brain tissues, like the nerve cells and the connections between them, which can give scientists an image of the numerous brain areas.

They found that typically, men's brains were larger. But women's brains had larger subregions of the cortex the cortical subregions are discrete parts of this particular brain area associated with memory, sensory input, learning, and making choices. Furthermore, there was a ton of variation in the sizes of different brain regions in guys; women's brains tended to be more comparable to one another. The research, which hasn't yet been peer-reviewed, was released in BioArXiv previously this month.

These findings aren't brand brand-new. But many neuroscience studies to date only looked at a sample size of a few hundred individuals. The thousands of brains here verify a lot of prior work. The simple fact that guys' brains had more distinctions among them fits with a ton of other evidence that appears to point toward males being more variable physically and psychologically, Stuart Ritchie, a psychologist and lead author of the paper, told Science. Likewise, it wasn't unexpected to find that ladies tended to have thicker cortices over all based upon prior findings (paywall).

The distinctions between women and men's brains were small enough that it d be impossible for researchers to identify an individual's sex by taking a look at his or her brain alone. Brain size and structure are attributes sort of like nose shape: they depend on a lot of different hereditary aspects, and can handle countless different types. And although a lot of men have bigger noses (and brains) than women, that's not always the case.

And it's essential to consider that different brain sizes and areas don't necessarily translate to actual behavioral distinctions, like intelligence. Our text is just about defining the distinctions, and we can't say anything about the reasons for those distinctions, Ritchie told New York Magazine. Different environmental and social factors play a big role in identifying the methods we believe and engage with one another.

Conclusion

Men depend on just one small area on the left side of the brain to complete the task, while the majority of women used parts in both sides of the brain. Nevertheless, both males and females sounded out the words similarly well, suggesting that there is more than one way for the brain to reach the same outcome. For instance, while ladies get stuck with a bad track record for checking out maps, it might just be that they orient to landmarks differently. And as for intelligence, average IQ ratings are the same for both women and men. With greater understanding of the structure of guys' and ladies' brains, he added, treatment of diseases affecting the brain could be improved through development of sex-specific medicines. Currently, scientists can't measure how much a person has male- or female-like patterns of brain connection. Another remaining question is whether the structural distinctions lead to differences in brain function, or whether differences in function result in structural changes.